"Katherine and Izzy provide the *couple lens*—offering long-needed, lived-experience expertise exploring and honoring both worlds  tips for individuals or their loved ones new to u ɪtal illness and distress. When I think back to my ʋ to live with a mental illness—well, I knew it as ɪ and it personally, I went searching or rather digg ɪfor- mation with accessible language and examples that I could use xpe- riences, rather than feeling isolated and engulfed in an illness. Katherine and Izzy—you provide the language to family and friends to talk about living life and recovery, giving them a sense of hope that families can thrive through these experiences."

> —**Chyrell D. Bellamy, PhD, MSW**, professor in the Yale University department of psychiatry, and director of the Yale Program for Recovery and Community Health

"Mental illness is common and often prolonged. While professionals provide important aspects of care and treatment, a substantial burden often remains with the affected persons. In this book, the authors share their extensive lived experience as someone with mental illness and her caregiver who addressed these many issues. The nine chapters are filled with knowledge and techniques critical to reducing illness experience and enhancing life."

> —**William Carpenter, MD**, professor emeritus at the University of Maryland Baltimore

"Mental illness challenges not only people struggling with symptoms and disabilities, but also their families and friends. This book is an elegant mix of hope and direction so caregiver and person with lived experience can partner toward recovery. The book is filled with practical information related to navigating psychiatric treatment, dealing with triggers, and forming a wellness plan. Along with her husband Izzy, Katherine tells a story of aspiration."

> —**Patrick Corrigan**, distinguished professor of psychology at the Illinois Institute of Technology where he directs the Center for Health Equity, Education, and Research

"I have spent my career studying and building knowledge about recovery from mental illness. Katherine and Izzy bring many of the principles in this field to life in their new book, *Loving Someone with a Serious Mental Illness*. Their practical and deeply personal guide offers a step-by-step approach to help individuals and caregivers navigate the complex journey toward recovery, making this book a vital resource for anyone facing similar challenges."

> —**Larry Davidson, PhD**, emeritus professor of psychiatry in the School of Medicine at the Yale University Program for Recovery and Community Health

"Nothing in our culture prepares us to become caregivers for someone we love who lives with serious mental illness. This book provides a hands-on blueprint for the challenges and trauma that devastate so many families. In concrete and compassionate storytelling, it teaches collaboration with your loved one plus caregiving for the caregiver. As a family peer supporter, this is a gift that brings sensitivity and confidence to the family in crisis."

—**John DeNatale**, father of sons living with serious mental illness, and NAMI Family-to-Family instructor

"In her latest book, patient advocate and recovery coach Katherine Ponte, along with her husband Izzy Goncalves, present a treasure trove of information for patients and their loved ones on how best to navigate the complexities and challenges they face while on the road to recovery from mental illness. Practical, readable, well researched and sourced, and infused with the wisdom of lived experience, this is a must-read for anyone living with (or caring for someone with) mental illness who strives for the best life possible."

—**Joseph F. Goldberg, MD**, clinical professor of psychiatry at the Icahn School of Medicine at Mount Sinai

"Katherine and Izzy have written a highly informative and digestible book in a relatable style from both a family member and consumer perspective. While very much grounded in science, it offers insightful and doable strategies for handling common challenges that arise in the everyday life of caring for and living with a serious mental illness. A must-read for families, consumers, and professionals alike. It has much to offer everyone."

—**Phyllis Solomon, PhD**, professor/associate dean for research in the School of Social Policy and Practice at the University of Pennsylvania

"Katherine and Izzy's book is a practical guide all families engaging with loved ones with mental health conditions should be able to access. As a parent of a child who developed a serious mental illness that led to his death, I believe deeply in the importance of resources that can help everyone navigate this journey and help ensure different, more hopeful outcomes. Katherine and Izzy's collaboration honors the expertise of both the individuals living with serious mental illness and their family caregivers, while delivering easy-to-understand information that is underpinned by the premise of hope for recovery and thriving."

—**Ken Zimmerman**, CEO of Fountain House, a national mental health nonprofit that empowers people living with serious mental illness through direct services, practice innovation, and policy change

Loving Someone with a Serious Mental Illness

Caring for Your Loved One and Yourself on the Journey to Mental Health Recovery

KATHERINE PONTE
IZZY GONCALVES

New Harbinger Publications, Inc.

Publisher's Note

This publication is designed to provide accurate and authoritative information in regard to the subject matter covered. It is sold with the understanding that the publisher is not engaged in rendering psychological, financial, legal, or other professional services. If expert assistance or counseling is needed, the services of a competent professional should be sought.

NEW HARBINGER PUBLICATIONS is a registered trademark of New Harbinger Publications, Inc.

New Harbinger Publications is an employee-owned company.

Copyright © 2025 by Katherine Ponte and Izzy Goncalves
New Harbinger Publications, Inc.
5720 Shattuck Avenue
Oakland, CA 94609
www.newharbinger.com

All Rights Reserved

Cover design by Amy Shoup

Acquired by Jed Bickman

Edited by Joyce Wu

Library of Congress Cataloging-in-Publication Data on file

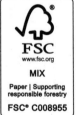

Printed in the United States of America

26   25   24

10   9   8   7   6   5   4   3   2   1   First Printing

We dedicate this book to each other and to the memory of our beloved Frenchie, Max, our loving companion from the start of our recovery journey, now with us in our hearts.

Contents

Foreword

In every life, there are situations that test the strength of our relationships, the depth of our compassion, and our capacity for understanding. One of the most profound challenges can be loving someone living with a serious mental illness. It is a journey that demands patience and resilience; yet it is also a journey that few are prepared for.

None of us is born knowing how to engage or communicate effectively with someone experiencing serious mental illness. Nor do we intuitively understand how to manage and maintain our own well-being while simultaneously adjusting to the unfamiliar and often unsettling new world in which we find ourselves.

In the absence of meaningful information, education, and support, family members and friends are winging it, making it up as we go along. As a result, we tend to say the very opposite of what the person needs to hear. The resulting stress and tension can erode relationships and wear thin the very fabric of families.

Izzy and Katherine understand these challenges intimately. They have lived through the highs and lows, the moments of clarity and confusion, and the trials that come with caring for someone living with mental illness. Their experiences have taught them that the road to recovery is paved by much more than merely good intentions.

Supporting a loved one with serious mental illness requires a foundation of knowledge, a variety of skills and tools, a boatload of patience, a support network who truly gets it, and the willingness and commitment to learn and grow. With access to information, education, and support, family and friends can better understand and engage the person they love to sustain and enhance critical relationships, benefitting the person living with mental illness, the people who love them, and society as a whole.

Family members frequently reach out to NAMI-NYC asking how to make their ill relative start or stop doing something. We are asking the wrong questions. In most cases, we cannot *make* an adult living with mental illness *do* anything. But when we start asking how we can improve our relationship, when we begin to explore what we can do differently that might alter how the other person responds or reacts to us, and when we shift how *we* show up—rather than try to change the way *they* do—the results can be transformative.

When family and friends have access to support and are able to make these efforts, outcomes for the person living with mental illness improve. We see fewer visits to emergency rooms, fewer in-patient hospitalizations, and increases in engagement with community mental health programs and services. Family support is a win-win-win.

I certainly don't mean to imply it will be easy. Unfortunately, in many cases, it can be a long and difficult journey. A roller coaster of ups and downs. Izzy and Katherine remind us that, while mental illness affects individuals and families differently, we are not alone. There is support on this journey, and together, we can develop the understanding and provide the emotional support needed to make a significant difference in our lives, their lives, and our shared relationships.

The strategies and techniques Izzy and Katherine share in this book, borne out of their journeys—separate and together—can help you separate your family member or friend from their illness, allowing you to love them and access the empathy and compassion to support them while simultaneously feeling however you may about their condition and how it affects them.

It is much better to be fighting together than fighting each other.

I believe this book will help countless individuals and families trying to navigate the challenges of serious mental illness. I encourage caregivers to pay particular attention to the discussion of self-care in addition to strategies for helping your loved one. It is as dangerous as it is easy to put yourself last. Mental illness can be isolating, not only for the person living with it, but also for the people who love them. Caregiver support can help you avoid burnout, help you develop appropriate boundaries and guard-rails, and provide you with actionable approaches and various outlets to take care of yourself along your journey. If you haven't dealt with mental illness yourself or through a family member or close friend, it can be difficult (if not impossible) to truly understand, to know what to say or how to be supportive. You may find it helpful to connect with others who understand what you're going through because they are going through something similar. The validation that comes with talking about what we are experiencing or how we are feeling and seeing others nodding because they truly understand cannot be overstated. This is the power of family support.

As you embark on this journey, remember every step you take toward understanding and compassion is a step toward healing and recovery—not only for your loved one but for you as well.

One in five of us lives with mental illness. The other four are our family, friends, neighbors, colleagues... We are all affected by mental illness.

And we are not alone.

—Matt Kudish, LMSW, MPA
Chief Executive Officer
National Alliance on Mental Illness of
New York City (NAMI-NYC)

Introduction

Our book is written by someone with serious mental illness (SMI), Katherine, and her spouse and caregiver, Izzy. We share strategies and tools for other families—loved ones with SMI and their caregivers—to navigate the challenges of SMI. These insights are based on the lessons we have learned in our over twenty-year journey with SMI—from the mistakes and lost opportunities to the constructive mindsets and collaboration that enabled us to reach recovery.

Katherine's Story

When Izzy and I met, we were both living our dreams. I was a lawyer and foreign legal consultant at the top law firm in Brazil, soon to pursue my MBA at one of the best business schools in the world. He was an associate at what many considered the top investment bank in the world. We both worked extremely hard and were proud of our humble roots. We were from Portuguese immigrant households, living parallel lives, seemingly perfect for each other. We were motivated to succeed and prove our worth for ourselves and our families. As partners who really understood and supported each other, it felt meant to be—we would be happy and might even accomplish more together. But that idyllic story would not play out as we imagined at the time.

While getting my MBA at Wharton, I faced a series of challenges that I could not have foreseen: academic stress, career uncertainty, a preoccupation with social injustice, family illness, and a sexual assault. I know now that together these factors triggered my severe bipolar I disorder with psychosis. That was the beginning of eighteen years of seeming loss—the life we planned but would not have—for my spouse and me. My mental illness journey over that time included several severe psychotic manic episodes resulting in three involuntary hospitalizations, long periods of deep depression with suicidal ideation, an arrest, and chronic unemployment. I was barely existing, hopeless, and seemingly helpless. At many times, I felt utterly alone. And so did my spouse.

Izzy and I both felt ashamed and embarrassed. We feared failure—specifically, to meet the goals we had imagined. And additionally, we were failing our relationship. Both of our lives were changed by my mental illness. Our roles were redefined, and this new reality threatened our plans and hopes. Husband and wife became caregiver and patient. We were not always united. We withdrew and isolated from others and each other. Instead of enjoying time together, he focused on maintaining calm and stability at home. He tried to contain the uncertainty that my illness had brought into our household, our relationship, and our prospects for success as a couple and as individuals.

I didn't want to accept this reality, so I resisted treatment. I didn't want the life depicted by the widespread stigma against people with SMI— to be viewed as crazy, defective, unstable, unable, and unemployable. I needed to take ownership of my illness to achieve lasting recovery. But I couldn't accept the identity of a person with SMI, or the stigma attached to it. And my treatment was not effective or suited to my needs. I had one psychiatrist who would fall asleep during our sessions and another one who told me that I would never get better—that my manic episodes would only become stronger and more frequent. Sadly, everyone else in my life seemed to think so as well.

My husband resented me for being passive about my treatment because my mental illness continued to threaten our stability. I resented the fact that his only concern about me was my illness, that he would seem to avoid me out of fear of a confrontation—we barely spoke to each other. I was expecting him to leave me. I thought he didn't love me anymore. We both lost hope.

Izzy's Story

I was a driven young man utterly devoted to my career and the success it promised. My plans assumed that I would have a smooth and happy family life. When Katherine's illness creeped into our lives, I was totally unprepared. Like Katherine, I initially didn't want to accept that we were a family with SMI, which could put our vision of success at risk. But I was ultimately forced to adapt to this new reality.

I resented that Katherine might be holding me back from achieving my goals. I had not signed up for this. I also felt like the object of Katherine's own resentment and outright anger. She blamed me for the times I'd called 911 and had her hospitalized. She said that I overreacted. Frankly, I didn't know if I had. What do you do when your wife descends into a full-blown psychosis, unable to sleep or contain her emotions—maybe running off across the city or darting from cabs? How far do you allow mania to escalate before calling 911? I didn't know. I also knew that many relationships didn't survive SMI—a frightening fact to contemplate.

These episodes were highly destructive for her and me. The lows were also silently devastating. They stopped her from addressing her illness, from living. In fact, I know now that those lows were potentially more life-threatening to her than I realized at the time.

I also didn't realize that all this was traumatic for me. I simply didn't have time or space to spend on my own emotions. I needed to grin and bear it. I numbed myself in order to survive. But I did hold out some hope—it may have seemed like blind hope—that we might get back on our path. It would take us longer to get there now, but we could still get there.

Ultimately, it was only after Katherine's third hospitalization that something changed.

Our Story

During that hospitalization, at my very lowest point in the psych ward, I (Katherine) saw a video of a person like me. They had experienced challenges with SMI similar to my own, but they had overcome them to live in recovery. I was no longer alone. I finally saw the possibility of recovery for me too. That flicker of hope allowed me and Izzy to imagine the possibilities of recovery—for both of us.

The journey was full of uncertainty. It required changes in my life, including in my treatment, which also introduced new risks. But I now had hope, which was incredibly empowering. I sought out and found more examples of peers living fulfilling lives with SMI. I found insight and support from their recovery journeys and shared my own. It helped guide me on my own path to recovery.

Although he supported me and held out hope of getting back on our path, Izzy had trouble adjusting to my transition and a resetting of our roles. He was still in survival mode, focused on maintaining calm. This created new challenges for us because our expectations and objectives grew apart. I resented that he seemed more interested in keeping me tame than allowing me to reclaim the true me. I had always been dynamic and driven before mental illness stole me. Now I had hope that I could be more like that person again. I had new motivation and energy to make a change.

But any change in my treatment created uncertainty and concern in Izzy, who worried that it might destabilize my mood and behavior, potentially triggering another episode. He was so afraid that, when I told him I had found a new psychiatrist, he threatened to divorce me if it triggered another manic episode. It was a statement made in understandable fear of the future.

But while there would be stumbles and pain along the way, we managed to overcome the challenges, through the guidance you'll learn in this book. And the risks I took to pursue recovery proved worthwhile.

My new psychiatrist, Joseph Goldberg, literally saved my life. It was the first time in sixteen years I felt a treatment provider really cared for me. He was not just concerned about treating my illness. More importantly, he understood what I truly needed was to gain my life back, the life I had lost to my mental illness. He created a new medication regimen that incorporated my goals. I would no longer be numbed and sedated by medication, which stunted my ability to achieve and live fully.

Izzy started to see results and realized that recovery was possible. Our expectations and objectives realigned. Our communication improved, and we finally became partners in the recovery journey. We were able to reach recovery only when we finally worked together with that shared goal. In the course of that work, we both slowly realized that it was possible to live a good life with mental illness.

I reached recovery about five years ago. What does it mean to live in recovery? To live in recovery is to live a full and meaningful life with mental illness. It does not mean to be cured of the illness, or to be symptom free. Also, it goes beyond merely treating symptoms, which is still one of the most pervasive treatment goals among clinicians. The SMI community is increasingly focused on recovery as an evolving treatment goal.

The odds of reaching mental health recovery can exponentially improve when caregivers—like you—and your loved ones work together to reach this shared goal. This book is for families with adult loved ones—in most cases a child, spouse, partner, sibling, or friend—with SMI. We wrote this book to help you, and your loved one, on this journey. We don't pretend to know your exact struggles, but our experiences with our own struggles may offer relevant insights and learnings.

Caregiving can be an isolating experience, but you are not alone. There are countless caregivers, in both families of origin and of choice, assisting the over fourteen million people who live with SMI in the US (SAMHSA 2021) Our book talks about what helped and could have helped us, so you can learn from our experience.

We acknowledge that we have been fortunate to have access to relatively good physical and mental health treatment. It goes without saying that people with SMI and their caregivers who find themselves disenfranchised from access to healthcare and other material resources face extraordinary additional challenges to pursue recovery. It's also true that, despite our access, treatment alone does not in and of itself guarantee recovery. Finding the healthcare providers who understand the meaning and importance of recovery in the broadest sense can be elusive. Still, the goal should always be recovery: reaching a place where your loved one and you with them can pursue a safe, dignified, and meaningful life.

The insight we will share with you is also based on the accounts of innumerable fellow peers, leading scholars like my wonderful mentor, Larry Davidson, and treatment providers who have greatly influenced my work. However, recovery is a highly individualized journey. What worked for us and for others may not work for you exactly, but some of it may. Finding out what works for you and your loved one may take considerable time, patience, and effort, but you must never give up. Our book shares various tools and perspectives that may be helpful to you along the way.

We wrote this book to give meaning and purpose to what we experienced. I (Katherine) strive to reach as many people as I can—particularly those who may be struggling the most, like psychiatric patients—through my peer support, writing, coaching, public speaking, and nonprofit work. I've noticed that the learnings of people with SMI are often unrecognized and unappreciated, and so I hope to impart what I've learned as a person living with SMI. We've also written this book to ensure that often-overlooked caregivers are included in the conversation around SMI. Izzy is a critical part of everything that happened to me and everything I do. And caregivers need ways to care for their loved ones and themselves.

In most families, the tendency is to live through episodes and set them aside, avoid speaking about them, because they can be just too painful to relive. Many people don't see these as learning opportunities. As a result, the same mistakes are repeated. Our goal in writing this book—and sharing the experience of a person with SMI along with their caregiver—is to help people with SMI and their caregivers avoid the same vicious cycle.

Finally, we also wrote this book because we have some regrets. We regret what we didn't know more about mental illness before it entered our relationship. We regret that we allowed mental illness to define us and our relationship. Unfortunately, so much of this experience is driven by stigma and stereotypes that only perpetuate SMI's baseless control over us. We regret that we isolated from each other instead of working together sooner. We regret that we struggled for so long when we didn't need to, if we had just known more.

We wrote this book to inform and empower you and the many other caregivers and loved ones who can benefit from our lessons learned—so that you can avoid these regrets. We hope to spare you some of the same uncertainties that prevented us from reaching recovery sooner. It doesn't have to be as hard for as long as it was for us.

Our book includes the essentials and the big picture. It shares strategies that will get your journey to recovery started, keep you on your path, and make you better and stronger to navigate the challenges and opportunities ahead. If recovery is not necessarily an objective for you and your loved one at the moment, we hope it will become one. No one book can cover all the situations you may encounter on your journey, but you may be able to apply learnings from the scenarios and strategies we describe.

We hope these insights can help lead you to the life you deserve. And in this work, we find tremendous meaning and purpose.

CHAPTER 1

Understanding Your Situation

This chapter helps you understand your loved one's condition and consider the impact of a diagnosis. It introduces various mental illnesses and their symptoms to help you and your loved one assess your situation so you can make positive change.

In the early stages of your loved one's mental health challenges, it's common to grapple with what's happening. Symptoms might initially be attributed to short-term stress, a topic explored in chapter 6, Identifying and Responding to Triggers. Stress, whether unusual or typical, can uncover a biological vulnerability, triggering mental health symptoms.

Once this trigger is activated, it becomes crucial for you, as a caregiver, to monitor the progression, staying vigilant for early warning signs—changes in eating or sleeping patterns, withdrawal from social interactions, unexplained physical discomfort, persistent worrying or guilt, and more. Recognizing these signs is vital for timely intervention.

It's important not to dismiss these signs, especially when they surface without an apparent cause. Don't underestimate internal triggers. As discussed in chapter 6, these are emotional reactions to past or present experiences that can lead to a spontaneous onset of symptoms or negative behaviors. Avoid assuming it's a passing phase or that symptoms will naturally fade away.

Recognizing warning signs is essential, because it allows you to intervene early, potentially leading to better outcomes. However, only a healthcare professional can provide a definitive diagnosis—a process that might be frustrating and time-consuming. Misdiagnoses are common. Differentiating between various mental health conditions can be challenging. This is especially true when someone has comorbidities (i.e., two or more psychiatric disorders that coincide), which is common and can create additional challenges for effective treatment and contribute to poorer outcomes.

Don't be surprised to experience shock and confusion when your loved one receives a diagnosis. This emotional upheaval prompts many caregivers to seek information. While online resources can be valuable, it's essential to consult reputable sources such as the Centers for Disease Control (CDC), Mayo Clinic, National Alliance on Mental Illness (NAMI), National Institute of Mental Health (NIMH), or Substance Abuse and Mental Health Services Administration (SAMHSA). Trusted friends and family who have experienced mental illness can also offer insight. A treatment provider is generally the best source of information.

According to SAMHSA (2021), SMI is defined as a "mental, behavioral, or emotional disorder resulting in serious functional impairment, which substantially interferes with or limits one or more major life activities." It commonly refers to bipolar disorder, major depressive disorder, and schizophrenia/schizoaffective disorder, but it may also include anxiety disorders, attention deficit disorders, borderline personality disorder, obsessive compulsive disorder, post-traumatic stress disorder, and more. Many SMIs share certain common symptoms to varying degrees, such as anxiety, agitation, psychosis, and more.

It's important to recognize that the experience of SMI will vary significantly with individual backgrounds and circumstances. A discussion of mental health must be adapted to these differences. These may include a consideration of race, ethnicity, gender (including gender identity and sexual orientation), faith, age, place of residence, being unhoused, relationship status, and much, much more.

In the sections that follow, and throughout this book, we focus on what many consider to be the most common SMIs, but many of the concepts and principles we describe likely have broad applicability to all SMIs.

Major Depressive Disorder

Major depressive disorder is the most prevalent SMI. Approximately 8 percent of US adults have experienced at least one major depressive episode (NIMH n.d.). Sadly, major depressive disorder often goes undetected and undertreated.

Symptoms

The primary indicator of a major depressive episode is a pervasive loss of interest or pleasure in nearly all activities. Other symptoms include persistent feelings of sadness, fatigue, changes in sleep patterns, changes in appetite, cognitive impairment, agitation, feelings of worthlessness or guilt, and suicidal thoughts or actions.

Distinguishing major depressive episodes from everyday depression that is linked to stressful life events is crucial. Major depressive episode symptoms can last *three months or longer* and can occur seemingly without cause. Major depressive disorder, also known as "unipolar depression," occurs when these down periods are not accompanied by high periods. Individuals with bipolar I, bipolar II, and schizophrenia commonly experience high rates of major depressive episodes.

How Caregivers Can Respond

One of the challenges you may encounter is that the depression causes your loved one to withdraw and isolate, hindering communication. At these times, they also ruminate on negative thoughts. You can try to listen and empathize. Instead of telling your loved one what you can do to help, ask if you can help them and how. You can offer suggestions or examples of how you may help, but do not insist on helping. Suggesting ways you can try to help may open the possibilities to your loved one, who may assume you are not willing to help with certain things.

Distraction is a great way to address depression. You can suggest activities and approaches as described further in the Wellness Plan in chapter 7. It can be toxic for your loved one to stay in bed or remain inactive. Gentle encouragement rather than criticism or ultimatums usually works best to encourage a loved one to mobilize themself.

Suicidality

Depression significantly elevates the risk of suicide. While predicting suicide remains unreliable, a history of depression and suicide attempts heightens the risk. You can play a critical role by opening conversations about suicide, which can be crucial in helping your loved one seek treatment and avoid a (or another) suicide attempt.

Some people may experience suicidal thoughts or behaviors because their underlying condition is getting worse. For others, longstanding or chronic suicidal thoughts may be a persistent condition that requires management but not emergency action.

How Caregivers Can Respond

For help with a suicidal crisis now, call 988 to reach the Suicide and Crisis Lifeline (in the US) or refer to the resources section of our book for more crisis lines.

People with SMI are at a higher risk of suicide. You must always take seriously suicidal statements, threats, or behaviors from your loved one. Don't dismiss comments about wanting to "kill myself" as your loved one just wanting attention. Talk about it. According to NIMH, "acknowledging and talking about suicide may reduce rather than increase suicidal thoughts" (n.d.). In fact, you might respond with something like "We have to take suicidal comments or behaviors with the utmost seriousness... What do you think you might do?" If your loved one is not sure that they can keep themself safe, you should ask them to seek immediate professional help by calling their doctor or 988 or appropriate emergency services. Direction from the treatment provider is critical to guide action. When in doubt, always call 988, especially if your loved one has engaged in self-harm now or in the past or is threatening to act on their suicidal comments.

It is far preferable to have a "safety plan" in place to address suicidal thoughts or statements before they come up. Ask your loved one how and whether they have proactively discussed the safety plan with their treatment provider. It is good self-care to assure that your mental health provider has an emergency contact to reach on your behalf as part of a safety plan.

Bipolar Disorder

Bipolar disorder causes significant shifts in mood, energy levels, thinking, and behavior during episodes. These episodes are often recurring. These episodes generally involve experiences of mania or depressions that vary in severity. Mood states stay relatively normal between episodes. This condition affects over 4 percent of the US population (NIMH n.d.), with the most common being bipolar I and bipolar II disorder. Bipolar II disorder entails a milder form of mania called hypomania. In both bipolar I and II disorder, significantly more time is spent in depression than mania/hypomania.

Phases

In one sense, bipolar disorder involves two main phases: highs and lows. However, on a deeper level these phases can be subdivided along a continuum as described below.

MANIA

People with bipolar I disorder experience mania, which is characterized by elevated mood, irritability, sleeplessness, and severe disturbances that impair functioning. Symptoms include rapid speech, increased restlessness, flight of ideas, distractibility, and exaggerated self-confidence. Psychotic features, like delusions and hallucinations, are prevalent in bipolar I disorder.

HYPOMANIA

Hypomania is a milder form of mania without psychosis. Bipolar I and II disorder both involve hypomania. When hypomanic, your loved one may exhibit elevated moods, heightened sociability, creativity, and productivity. People with bipolar disorder often enjoy hypomanic states, while fearing the descent into depression. As a result, during hypomanic periods, treatment and medication adherence may be challenging, as your loved one may resist suppressing hypomania.

Hypomania in and of itself does not require hospitalization. However, manic episodes often start as hypomania, reinforcing the important role you can have in preventing this progression.

MIXED FEATURES

Episodes with mixed features involve symptoms of depression and mania or hypomania simultaneously. These episodes are more challenging to diagnose, and recovery takes longer compared to episodes of pure hypo/mania. Over half of depressed-phase bipolar disorder patients exhibit mixed features (Goldberg et al. 2009).

Anosognosia

Anosognosia, a lack of awareness of being ill, commonly occurs with bipolar I disorder, especially during mania (Ghaemi, Stoll, and Pope 1995). This lack of insight is not mere denial but a deeply ingrained, involuntary unawareness of symptoms. Understandably, lacking awareness of the condition contributes to nonadherence to treatment.

Suicidality

People with bipolar disorder face high suicide rates. Suicide risk, which is linked to depression severity, is particularly high in the initial years of the condition (Angst et al. 2002). This pattern reinforces the importance of early treatment.

For help with a suicidal crisis, see above for more guidance.

How Caregivers Can Respond

The appropriate response to bipolar disorder will depend largely on which phase your loved one is in.

MANIA

It is crucial for caregivers to understand and address mania. During a manic episode, your loved one may be unaware of their behavior, especially when they experience psychosis.

Trying to communicate with your loved one during these periods is critical. Listen attentively, empathize with their emotions, and avoid arguments. If conversations turn unproductive or agitated, give your loved one space. Be mindful of their voice and body language for cues about their state of mind. You should also try to minimize environmental stimulation. If your loved one is on medication, gently inquire if they've taken it— without accusations. While ensuring your safety, resist imposing threats or physical restraint. It may be necessary to take emergency measures if your loved one poses a danger to themself or others, including you, as discussed in chapter 5, Navigating Psychiatric Treatment.

HYPOMANIA

It can be important to recognize the delicate balance that your loved one may be navigating between the pleasure of hypomania and the fear of depression. Try to approach this situation with empathy.

If your loved one is hypomanic, they may not readily share that they're experiencing symptoms or their consequences, such as excessive spending or risky decision-making. They may even attempt to conceal their behavior in order to preserve the often-elated state brought by hypomania and avoid slipping back into depression. You should carefully word your questions to help clarify the difference between normal behavior and emerging hypomania. It's a delicate process, as directly pointing out their state may trigger resistance. Expressing curiosity is a helpful approach. Encourage open discussion about their feelings using listening techniques discussed in chapter 8, Talking About Mental Illness. Gently discuss potential outcomes of their behavior, offering support to help them achieve their objectives while maintaining close contact. Reassure them that you're glad they're feeling well but express a desire to ensure they can maintain this state.

ANOSOGNOSIA

It may be very frustrating if your loved one seems to deny their condition, particularly when the signs of mania or psychosis are clear to you. However, anosognosia may render them genuinely unaware of their symptoms. Challenging their understanding is often unhelpful. Maintain a stance of curiosity and compassion. The listening techniques discussed more in chapter 8, Talking About Mental Illness may help you. Find common ground and empathize with their distress instead of disputing their beliefs. Establishing and maintaining trust may leave your loved one more willing to collaborate on treatment adherence. If the situation becomes combative, step back and suggest revisiting the discussion at another time.

Psychosis

Psychosis spans a range of symptoms that disrupt an individual's connection with reality. Recognizing these symptoms early is vital. Studies indicate that between fifteen and one hundred people out of one hundred thousand develop psychosis annually (NIMH n.d.). Psychosis most commonly occurs in people with schizophrenia and bipolar I disorder and is frequently triggered by substance use. Since psychosis often starts in young adulthood, early identification and intervention is possible and can prevent full-fledged psychotic episodes, improving long-term outcomes. There are early intervention programs for psychosis across the country.

Schizophrenia, bipolar disorder, and major depressive disorder are often accompanied by psychosis as a symptom. Delusions and auditory hallucinations are prevalent in people with schizophrenia, with an estimated 80 to 90 percent experiencing delusions (Columbia University Department of Psychiatry 2019). Prevalence rates range from 50 to 75 percent in bipolar I disorder (Elowe et al. 2022), while up to 19 percent of major depressive disorder cases involve psychotic features (Ruggero et al. 2011).

Symptoms

Psychosis typically involves delusions—continuous, false fixed beliefs—and hallucinations—sensory experiences (e.g., seeing or hearing things)—that occur without typical external stimuli. Delusions can be persecutory, grandiose, or guilt-related, depending on the SMI:

- Persecutory delusions are the most common type for people with schizophrenia. They are marked by extreme paranoia, fear in ordinary situations, and constant seeking of safety.

- Delusions of grandeur are most common for people with bipolar I disorder. Grandiose delusions involve beliefs of excessive power, wealth, or intelligence.

- Delusions of guilt are most common for people with major depressive disorder. These involve unwarranted and extreme feelings of remorse, low self-worth, and feeling that punishment is deserved for some perceived transgression.

Hallucinations can involve auditory or visual experiences. Auditory, or sound, hallucinations are the most common. They involve hearing sounds that aren't real, such as music, footsteps, banging, and people's voices. Visual hallucinations involve seeing objects, shapes, lights, people, or animals that are not present. Hallucinations in the absence of delusions or other psychiatric symptoms may sometimes point to a non-psychiatric or neurological explanation, such as epilepsy or toxic environmental exposures. Possible non-psychiatric causes such as these require a careful medical workup.

Belief Conviction

Belief conviction means that individuals are certain about their beliefs, even in the face of contrary evidence. This lack of awareness of what is real is a defining feature of psychosis. Because a delusion is a false fixed belief, you cannot talk someone out of it.

Comorbidity

Substance misuse can worsen or trigger psychosis, especially in schizophrenia or bipolar disorder. People with mental illness, including psychosis, are generally more likely to misuse substances compared to the general population. They are more likely to use cannabis, linked to earlier onset of psychosis in those with genetic risk factors (Urits et al. 2020). Cognitive impairment often accompanies SMIs, posing additional barriers to recovery and causing disability.

How Caregivers Can Respond

How you should respond depends on whether your loved one has yet been diagnosed and has a treatment plan. Seek a professional evaluation at the onset of symptoms. Once a diagnosis is established, follow the treatment plan.

If you lack experience with this type of behavior, avoid questioning or challenging your loved one's perspective. Instead, acknowledge their emotions, highlighting observations of distress or confusion. Be a consistent presence. If psychotic symptoms escalate, know the doctor's recommendations, when to call for safety concerns, and be aware of potential medication nonadherence. Approach questions about medication use empathically, expressing genuine concern for their well-being.

Schizophrenia

Schizophrenia is a poorly understood and stigmatized mental illness, affecting less than 1 percent of the US population (NAMI n.d.). Schizophrenia is mainly a disorder of thinking and perception.

Symptoms

Symptoms of schizophrenia encompass positive (exaggerated thoughts or perceptions) and negative (loss of normal function) aspects. Positive symptoms include delusions (e.g., thinking people are spying on you when they are not), hallucinations (e.g., hearing voices that are not there), disorganized thinking (e.g., expressing ideas that incoherently flow from one to the next), and abnormal motor behavior (e.g., posturing, making odd gestures or mannerisms). Negative symptoms include diminished emotional expression (called "flat affect") and avolition (having no motivation), which significantly impact social functioning. Cognitive impairment is also prevalent in schizophrenia, further complicating overall treatment. Emotional expression affects verbal and nonverbal cues, causing potential communication issues. Anosognosia is prevalent in schizophrenia.

Suicidality

Suicidality is common among people with schizophrenia. This risk is highly related to negative symptoms and a demoralized sense of life and purpose. It also sometimes occurs from hallucinations (e.g., commands to hurt oneself).

For help with a suicidal crisis, see above.

How Caregivers Can Respond

We discussed above how to respond to psychosis and other positive symptoms associated with schizophrenia.

For information on treating positive symptoms, please refer to the previous section on psychosis. Negative symptoms, such as avolition as well as cognitive impairment, are admittedly challenging to address. In general, you should acknowledge specific challenges faced by your loved one and express a desire to help them. When unsure, ask your loved one for their ideas, proposing options while being aware that their symptoms may leave them feeling unsure or unable to generate ideas. It is often more important to be a supporter than a problem solver. This is a useful rule of thumb for many other situations as well.

Schizoaffective Disorder

Schizoaffective disorder combines features of schizophrenia and mood disorders. At times, your loved one may experience significant manic or depressive episodes, or both, with psychosis, and at other times, experience persistent psychosis with no mood symptoms. The patient experience is between that of schizophrenia and bipolar.

Symptoms Across All SMIs

Agitation

Agitation, defined as excessive motor activity linked to inner tension, can escalate to nonproductive behaviors. It is also often linked with irritability. Agitation is prevalent in bipolar disorder and schizophrenia, where it can be associated with delusions and command hallucinations. While aggression is not a core feature, increasing agitation severity may lead to violent tendencies. It's crucial to recognize that the majority of those with SMI are not violent, more often being victims than perpetrators of violent crime.

How caregivers can respond: You can learn about and help your loved one practice self-care strategies, which are essential for preventing agitation. Learn about de-escalation techniques, detailed in chapter 4, Supporting Your Loved One on the Treatment Journey, which you can employ to manage your loved one's agitation.

Anxiety

Anxiety can be experienced as a distinct symptom without a formal anxiety diagnosis or as part of a specific anxiety diagnosis like panic disorder. It may also result from medication side effects or withdrawal from missed doses or substance use (e.g., withdrawal). Anxiety disorders often coexist with major depressive disorder, bipolar disorder, and schizophrenia, impacting treatment outcomes. People with anxiety disorders may experience intense worry, physical symptoms, and panic attacks, which significantly affect daily life.

Common signs of anxiety include restlessness, rapid heart rate, trembling, and sweating. Treatment may involve medications with antianxiety properties. Sometimes separate medications like antidepressants or sedatives may be necessary. There are many behavioral techniques to help manage or prevent flares of anxiety.

How caregivers can respond: Never invalidate or dismiss your loved one's anxiety. Recognize anxiety is not something they control. Caregivers can be reassuring and emphasize their supportive presence without disputing whether feeling anxious is justified. Activities and distraction techniques, such as going for a walk, can help alleviate anxiety.

Cognitive Impairments

Cognitive impairments are difficulties in processing information, including attention, focus, memory, and the ability to plan, organize, and manipulate information. All SMIs involve some degree of cognitive impairment. Some medicines, such as sedative hypnotics or antihistamines, can also cause cognitive side effects. These effects are considered most significant in schizophrenia, and unfortunately, they may progress over time. In bipolar disorder, cognitive impairment is believed to be more limited, affecting areas like attention, verbal memory, and executive functioning. Major depressive disorder often exhibits pronounced issues with attention and concentration due to the severity of depression, impacting academic or work performance. Moreover, subjective cognitive complaints sometimes reflect mood or anxiety symptoms rather than true, objective cognitive deficits. Many experts argue that cognitive problems in SMIs are often underestimated, hindering recovery even when mood or psychotic symptoms are addressed effectively.

How caregivers can respond: Recognize cognitive symptoms, like diminished memory and attention. Encourage your loved one to work on strategies for cognitive deficits. These may include non-medication treatments, like cognitive remediation, discussed in our Navigating Psychiatric Treatment chapter (5). Gently remind your loved to engage in assigned cognitive exercises.

Avolition

Avolition—a significant reduction in self-initiated, purposeful activities—may hinder many aspects of living. People with avolition may spend extended periods disinterested in work or social engagements. Unlike procrastination or laziness, avolition involves a genuine struggle to muster the emotional or physical energy needed for tasks. These challenges may lead to a sense of paralysis. Avolition is prevalent in SMIs.

How caregivers can respond: Compassion and empathy are crucial when responding to avolition. You should avoid judgment, recognizing avolition as a symptom, not a character trait. Express concern, offer support, and brainstorm small steps with your loved one to overcome this challenge. Emphasize that avolition is temporary and not their fault.

Substance Use

Substance use disorders (SUDs) often co-occur with SMIs. Nearly 50 percent of people with an SMI also experience a SUD (SAMHSA 2023).

SUDs complicate relationships and treatment approaches. You may find yourself negotiating with a loved one who is ambivalent about addiction recovery. Establishing rules and boundaries, encouraging attendance at support meetings, and considering intervention may be necessary, even when met with ambivalence. Some people use substances to self-medicate symptoms such as depression or anxiety, but others use substances because they produce reinforcing pleasurable states, and are abusable. Don't automatically assume all substance use is "just" self-medication; there may be a need for separate addiction or recovery treatment.

How caregivers can respond: If you suspect substance use, try to foster an open dialogue. Express concern to your loved one without accusing them. Balance care without appearing controlling or disciplinarian. Try to address your concerns collaboratively rather than coercively.

This chapter provided an introduction to various mental illnesses and their symptoms to help you and your loved one assess your situation so you can make positive change. The next chapter introduces the concept of recovery—the goal of the positive change that you and your loved one can work toward.

CHAPTER 2

Pursuing Recovery

Recovery is possible. It's actually common. Up to 65 percent of people living with SMI will experience partial to full recovery based on their symptoms and functioning (Davidson et al. 2008).

Knowing that recovery is probable—that you can live the life you want—is the single greatest motivator for your loved one to get well. They'll very likely take ownership of their illness and—with your support—do the hard work necessary to reach recovery.

This chapter introduces key recovery principles and strategies. It emphasizes the importance of hope and underscores the person-driven nature of recovery, urging you and your loved one to be actively involved in the healing process. It also emphasizes the importance of recognizing trauma, leveraging strengths, fostering responsibility and self-respect, and challenging stigma. If your loved one is not yet in recovery, the chapter addresses challenges like delayed diagnoses and self-sabotage. It concludes by discussing relapse, emphasizing that setbacks do not erase overall progress.

Defining Recovery

Recovery can have different formal and informal meanings. According to the work of leading mental illness recovery scholar Dr. Larry Davidson, also referencing the work of Professor Mike Slade (2009), there are two main types of recovery. There's "recovery from" or "clinical recovery" and there's "in recovery" or "personal recovery" (Davidson, Roe, and Tondora 2020), as described below.

Davidson and Roe (2009) provide the following definitions of both types of recovery:

"[Clinical] recovery from serious mental illnesses involves the amelioration of symptoms and the person's returning to a healthy state following onset of the illness. This definition is based on explicit criteria of levels of signs, symptoms, and deficits associated with the illness and identifies a point at which remission may be said to have occurred."

"Remission" has been defined to mean a reduction in psychiatric symptoms (such as problems with sleep, energy, and motivation) to the point that they are no more than minimally present. It's distinct from being "stable." "Stable" is used to mean that symptoms are not changing or are adequately controlled. For example, the patient's condition is not deteriorating but they may not yet be improving.

As opposed to clinical recovery, recovery from serious mental illness or personal recovery refers primarily to a person diagnosed with a serious mental illness reclaiming his or her right to a safe, dignified, and personally meaningful and gratifying life in the community while continuing to have a mental illness. It emphasizes self-determination and such normative life pursuits as education, employment, sexuality, friendship, spirituality, and voluntary membership in faith and other kinds of communities beyond the limits both of the disorder and of the mental health system, and consistent with the person's own goals, values, and preferences. (Davidson and Roe 2009)

Another widely cited definition of personal recovery describes it as a "deeply personal, unique process of changing one's attitudes, values, feelings, goals, skills and/or roles," and "a way of living a satisfying, hopeful, and contributing life even with the limitation caused by illness. Recovery involves the development of new meaning and purpose in one's life as one grows beyond the catastrophic effects of mental illness" (Anthony 1993).

Many aspects of these common definitions of recovery overlap. Clinical recovery and personal recovery are not mutually exclusive. In fact, clinical recovery is often, but not always, required to achieve personal recovery. Pursuing personal recovery also often requires that we achieve some stability—a consistent period of wellness—first. But recovery scholars often point out the value of pursuing personal recovery even when still symptomatic. Put simply, encourage your loved one not to wait for their symptoms to stop before they strive to achieve personal life goals.

In fact, because work and social activities can enhance one's sense of self-worth and self-efficacy, pursuing meaningful activities may facilitate recovery. Be careful not to discourage your loved one's aspiration simply because they're not in remission. With SMIs, remission can be elusive. Individuals often struggle with residual symptoms. Recovery in some ways demands they find ways to enhance coping and management and not allow symptoms to overwhelm life goals.

While clinical recovery has been the traditional focus of healthcare providers the emerging recovery model emphasizes a sense of meaning and purpose based on individual priorities and values over symptom relief. It focuses on strengths, in contrast to clinical recovery's focus on disorders, symptoms, and deficits.

The emerging model recognizes recovery as a practical, achievable outcome in which functioning and symptom levels improve over time. To reach recovery, you harness your strengths, resources, and sources of support. It requires hard work, but the payoff can be invaluable.

This book is mostly about personal recovery. When we refer to recovery, it is generally to personal recovery. However we define recovery, hope is central to reaching it. And there is reason to hope. You're here, working through this book. You and your loved one are engaged in the project of working to improve their life, and there are many skills and tools you can learn to help yourselves along the way.

If Your Loved One Has Not Yet Reached Recovery

If your loved one is not yet in recovery, or if you've struggled on this journey, know that you're not alone. It's sobering to realize this, but only 65 percent of adults with SMI receive any treatment at all (NAMI n.d.), and the average time of symptom onset to treatment is eleven years (NAMI n.d.).

What might explain these statistics? Reasons include difficulty getting a diagnosis and reluctance to recognize a condition because of stigma surrounding mental health conditions. Nonadherence to treatment, driven by factors like adverse medication reactions or a lack of belief in recovery, is also common. Self-sabotage, where individuals may undermine their progress due to fear of failure or relapse, is another obstacle.

Sometimes, despite caregivers' best efforts, loved ones may resist treatment. In such cases, caregivers may need to step back and allow them to confront the depths of their illness, hoping it will motivate their loved ones to take accountability for their recovery. Regardless of the challenges, maintaining hope and perseverance is essential, as the journey to recovery is ongoing and may involve setbacks. By working together, caregivers and loved ones can enhance the chances of success in the recovery process. The following principles of recovery can provide you with a firm foundation for working together with your loved one to pursue recovery.

Principles of Recovery

For all of us, pursuing and maintaining a meaningful life require staying well. What constitutes a meaningful life depends on the person. For some, it may mean a job; for others, it may mean better relationships with friends and family, or parenthood. You can work with your loved one to help identify what will motivate them to work to reach their best selves. For me (Katherine), it was working full time, being more active, and having better relationships. Whatever you and your loved one come up with, it'll be a powerful motivating force to maintain healthy behaviors and manage risks to your loved one's mental health.

Experience is the best teacher of what works and doesn't work, and it takes time, patience, and perseverance to figure out what works best. Still, there are some general principles that can guide us. SAMHSA has identified ten guiding principles of recovery (2012): hope, person-driven, many pathways, holistic, peer support, relational, culture, addresses trauma, strengths /responsibility, and respect. In the sections that follow, we'll explore each of these principles along with our suggestions on how you can support your loved one on the path to recovery.

PRINCIPLE 1: HOPE

All these principles can help someone reach recovery, but the most important for many is hope. Recovery is rarely achieved without hope. Its power cannot be overestimated.

Hope is the belief that a better future is possible. To start pursuing this possibility, we need to accept our mental illness. We must also accept that we need to make efforts to reach recovery and that it will be hard but worthwhile. This is the starting point for recovery, for your loved one and for you. Instilling hope may be especially difficult for loved ones who have struggled with depression, where a sense of hopelessness can sometimes become pervasive. Your loved one needs to find and keep hope, and you, and their other caregivers, must also have this hope so you can provide and foster hope in them. The circle of hope among supporters and the supported can be a very powerful driver of progress toward recovery. It can provide your loved one the motivation and conviction to persist and overcome challenges when they arise.

How hopeful do you think your loved one is right now? It's okay if the answer is "not very" or "not always." But it's useful to begin exploring how hopeful your loved one feels right now, how that sense of hope might be bolstered, and how you can communicate that hope to your loved one. This way you can stimulate and sustain their hope for the future. Crucially, that hope cannot be shallow. It should be grounded in acceptance of your loved one's experience and challenges.

Below are tips for communicating with your loved one to achieve hope. See chapter 8 for a more detailed discussion on how to talk about mental illness:

- Validate their feelings and empathize with their experience

- Maintain emotional balance, avoiding excessive displays of emotion

- Express unwavering belief in your loved one's capacity to achieve recovery, despite past challenges

- Sustain hope for their future, even during difficult times, as your optimism can be a powerful motivator

- Ensure healthcare providers maintain hope for your loved one's recovery, recognizing that treatment responses vary

- Support their dreams and assist in finding pathways to achieve them

- Focus on possibilities rather than limitations when discussing life with mental illness

- Celebrate both small and significant achievements without excessive surprise

- Encourage self-forgiveness and frame past mistakes as learning opportunities

- Commit to fighting alongside them in their journey toward recovery

PRINCIPLE 2: PERSON-DRIVEN

Recovery isn't handed to those with mental illness. We must seek and pursue our recovery, often by changing our behaviors and priorities across many dimensions of our lives. Your loved one must recognize their role in this process, learning from others' journeys and engaging with treatment providers to tailor a recovery plan. Their autonomy in this process is crucial for sustained progress.

What does all this mean for you, as your loved one's caregiver? A caregiver can significantly influence the experience of their loved one. Often, you're in a position of "seniority" or "responsibility" for your loved one. How do you balance your influence as a caregiver with giving your loved one space to exercise the control and ownership required to embrace treatment and pursue recovery? Below are some tips to exercise a healthy level of influence while promoting your loved one's self-determination:

- Empower your loved one by allowing them to make choices in their life

- Encourage their control over treatment, career, and relationships, offering guidance as needed

- Assist in crafting goals that are S.M.A.R.T. (Drucker 1954):

  - Specific—elaborating a single action

  - Measurable—progress should be easy to gauge

  - Achievable—something your loved one can feasibly accomplish in the time you've agreed to together

  - Reasonable—within reach

- Timely—goals your loved one can achieve in a reasonable timeframe, with a clear start and end point

- Remind them of their intrinsic worth and past achievements

- Avoid statements implying a decline in their capabilities

- Foster belief in their dreams and abilities

- Encourage them to pursue ambitious goals while staying realistic

- Remove unnecessary barriers to their aspirations

For more details on how to implement these ideas in your daily life, see chapter 7.

PRINCIPLE 3: MANY PATHWAYS

People experiencing mental illness have individual needs, strengths, weaknesses, and experiences that will influence their recovery journey. These conditions will lead and require your loved one to pursue their own pathway to recovery—their own unique combination of behavioral changes, treatments, and services. You and your loved one may work to access recovery through unique uses of clinical treatment, medication, therapy, support from friends and family, and peer support.

You'll also have to adjust along the way to address setbacks and new challenges, incorporate lessons learned, and ensure that those in your loved one's support network are being constructive and helpful. We should all, loved ones and caregivers alike, appreciate that recovery is not linear. There will be challenges, strains, and uncertainty along the way, which will require resilience and a supportive environment.

As a caregiver, you'll work with your loved one to identify, utilize, and build their strengths, resourcefulness, and resilience. Below are tips for helping your loved one plan their recovery journey:

- Help your loved one assemble and understand information about different strategies to pursue recovery, using sources that are well researched and shown to be effective

- Develop a schedule of specific objectives and goals

- Help your loved one assess their current state to set near-term and longer-term expectations

- Ensure your loved one is committed to seeking recovery— ultimately, it's up to them to reach recovery

- Discuss practical, actionable steps to achieve your loved one's recovery goals

- Make a plan to address or cope with specific personal weaknesses and obstacles that may arise as they pursue their goals

- Discuss calculated risk taking—decisions that could be beneficial but may also involve higher risk of failure or setback

- Let your loved one learn from their setbacks when they experience them; they inevitably will have setbacks at some point—we all do

- Work with others in your loved one's network to support and advance their efforts

- Remind your loved one that recovery is a journey, not a destination

PRINCIPLE 4: HOLISTIC

Recovery encompasses mental, physical, emotional, spiritual, and social aspects of life. Your loved one's journey toward recovery involves reevaluating daily activities, interactions, and self-care practices. Together, you must design a plan that aligns with their unique needs and priorities, integrating diverse tools and resources. These options include medical care, traditional and alternative therapy, community engagement, peer and social resources, and friends and family support.

As a caregiver, you can play an essential role promoting and supporting the wide range of opportunities for your loved one to improve their quality of life. Below are tips for helping your loved one improve their life holistically:

- Discuss different dimensions of life and prioritize those crucial to recovery as physical, intellectual, financial, environmental, spiritual, social, occupational, and emotional (Swarbrick 2012), as discussed in the Wellness Plan chapter (7)

- Research and share local resources for improving various aspects of life

- Work together to create a holistic wellness plan

- Assist in scheduling and attending appointments to access necessary services

PRINCIPLE 5: PEERS AND ALLIES

Support from peers and allies is invaluable in the recovery process. Peers with lived experiences can offer practical and relatable insights and inspiration, countering isolation and providing motivation. Engaging with peers can also be a source of meaning and purpose for your loved one if they can learn to share and help peers with their own insights.

Which sources of support from peers and allies have you helped your loved one secure? Which would you and your loved one like to secure? Below are tips for helping your loved access the benefits of peer support:

- Help identify opportunities for peer connections

- Seek out materials that recount different people's lived experiences with mental illness and recovery, like memoirs or other first-person accounts

- Assemble and share information on local Clubhouses (Clubhouse International is an organization dedicated to helping people experiencing mental illness find and build communities, or Clubhouses, in their area to encourage and support their recovery—one example is Fountain House in New York)

- Assemble and share information on local support groups— say, through a local NAMI affiliate or Depression and Bipolar Support Alliance (DBSA) support group

- Where more intensive care is needed, consider helping your loved one enroll in an outpatient program, which includes group treatment

- Explore opportunities where therapy is offered in a group format, such as cognitive behavioral therapy (CBT) and DBT (dialectical behavioral therapy) groups

- Encourage your loved one to give back to their peers to make them feel connected to the community and give them meaning and purpose (it can be small-scale—for instance, friends or peers experiencing the same or similar things, with whom your loved one maintains a supportive friendship, or volunteer opportunities your loved one can take advantage of to contribute to their community)

PRINCIPLE 6: RELATIONSHIPS AND SOCIAL NETWORKS

Positive relationships with friends and family members are crucial for sustained recovery. Surround your loved one with supportive people who appreciate the positivity your loved one can bring to themself and others. Encourage your loved one to develop a social network of peers who can envision living a life full of purpose and meaning. You may want to encourage your loved one to try to limit interactions with people who are discouraging, stigmatizing, or otherwise unhealthy in their influence on your loved one.

Below are tips for helping your loved experience supportive relationships:

- Again, it can start with you. Support your loved one to the greatest extent possible. Be an example to other people in their network.

- Encourage other family members to offer your loved one support.

- Explore opportunities—gatherings, group events—for your loved one to connect with others.

- Accompany your loved one to group events.

- You might, with the permission of your loved one, reach out to old friends and encourage them to reconnect with your loved one. Confirm with your loved one what details they are comfortable with you sharing.

- Work with your loved one to assess which of their relationships may be making their recovery harder, not easier. And have a conversation about what might be done about such relationships. Does your loved one need to set better boundaries regarding what they do and don't want this person to talk about or do? Encourage your loved one to limit the amount of time they spend around anyone who is discouraging. Might it be best for the relationship to end altogether?

PRINCIPLE 7: CULTURAL BACKGROUND AND INFLUENCE

Cultural background significantly influences mental health experiences and treatment preferences. It is important to work with healthcare professionals who appreciate and are sensitive to your loved one's cultural background. They may be better able to address your loved one's specific concerns and influences and provide more individualized patient assessment and treatment.

If your loved one belongs to an underrepresented community, it may be even more challenging to find treatment that is sensitive to their unique challenges. Below are tips for helping your loved one find care that is sensitive to their background:

- Discuss culturally competent care with your loved one and their treatment provider

- Identify and assemble information on examples of people from underrepresented communities living with mental illness

- Stress the strengths of diverse communities

- Seek out support groups such as those offered by some NAMI affiliates

PRINCIPLE 8: ADDRESSING TRAUMA

Traumatic events (e.g., violence, abuse, disaster) can have negative emotional repercussions that can contribute to mental health or substance use issues. Recovery requires acknowledging and coping with these traumas with support from professionals, peers, and family.

As a caregiver, you may often ask what caused your loved one's mental illness. While trauma can sometimes trigger the emergence of mental health symptoms, many experts believe that trauma is more likely to do so when, for a given individual, there is a pre-existing biological vulnerability to mental illness. This concept is the basis of the so called "diathesis-stress" model originally described by Zubin and Spring (1977). Trauma can aggravate the recovery process from mental illness, often involves sensitive work, and must be done with care, but you can work with your loved one to help them identify and understand their traumas.

Below are tips for helping yourself and your loved one better understand and address traumatic experiences:

- Identify possible traumatic events such as adverse childhood experiences, which according to the CDC (2024b), may include experiencing violence, abuse, or neglect; witnessing violence; having a family member attempt or die by suicide; and growing up in a household with substance use problems, untreated mental health problems, and instability.

- Discuss traumatic events your loved one may have endured and how those experiences may influence their experiences with mental health. Validate their experience.

- Be prepared to openly discuss trauma with healthcare providers, as your past experiences may impact treatment.

- Acknowledge the potential trauma of experiences related to the illness itself and encourage sensitivity in peers and your support network. Note that involuntary hospitalizations are one of the most traumatic experiences your loved one can experience while symptomatic.

- Highlight that often people find strength and resilience in the face of trauma, a circumstance known as post-traumatic growth (PTG). You can foster this growth in your loved one by recognizing the strengths they may show in bearing them. See chapter 6, Identifying and Responding to Triggers, for more.

PRINCIPLE 9: RECOGNIZING STRENGTHS AND RESPONSIBILITY

Recovery requires taking personal responsibility and ownership while leveraging support from family, friends, and communities. Taking responsibility can be a powerful source of strength and motivation for your loved one in their recovery.

Below are tips for helping your loved one access their own strengths as well as the resources available within their network:

- Help identify and address support needs, strengthening existing networks and building new ones as necessary

- Encourage your loved one to take ownership of their recovery and advocate for their needs

- Help a loved one self-advocate for their needs and concerns

- Show personal examples of advocacy in the mental health community through participation in organizations such as NAMI

PRINCIPLE 10: RESPECT

Your loved one must, with your help, accept that they deserve recovery and believe that they can do the work required; this acceptance is a form of self-respect. Also, it takes great courage to confront the challenges of mental illness—and often, these challenges are imposed on us by society, by stigma. So, those of us who do not experience mental illness must also show respect for this recovery, and for the rights of people with mental illness to social inclusion.

As a caregiver, ensuring that your loved one feels respect starts with you. Don't let bias and stigma, your own or others', get in the way of recovery. You can make sure your loved one recognizes that they should respect themself and deserve respect from others.

Below are tips for helping your loved one feel the respect that may be essential to motivating recovery:

- Assist your loved one in accepting their mental illness and recognizing their inherent worth beyond their condition

- Challenge stigma and biases that may hinder your loved one's recovery journey

- Respect your loved one's autonomy and choices, even when you disagree

Life Can Be Better After Recovery

Mental illness can be very difficult and disruptive, but it can also allow you and your loved one to gain a deeper appreciation of what's important in life. This awareness can lead many of us, both people with mental illness and caregivers, to reexamine our previous lifestyles, career choices, relationships, values, and dreams. The coping strategies and tools that you and your loved one develop to respond to triggers will better position you to pursue the relationships, work, and activities that provide fuller meaning to your lives.

Of course, you and your loved one may not yet have reached this stage. Your loved one may still be struggling with the challenges of mental illness. If so, stay hopeful for the possibility of recovery and the growth that can come out of their difficulties. And do all you can to advocate that your loved one pursue the avenues that may lead them toward recovery.

A Note on Relapse

Relapse, if it happens, may be one of the most discouraging times for your loved one. They may feel they've lost all the gains they made to get well, and they'll need to start over—without realizing they'll be starting over from a place of experience. In such moments, remind your loved one that relapse is always possible, and that doesn't mean that recovery is not ultimately achievable, no matter how many times a person has relapsed.

Moving Forward

In this chapter, you gained insights into fundamental principles of and strategies for mental health recovery. We addressed the importance of not just symptom reduction but also seeking a fulfilling life. Hope is essential to motivate and support your loved one and you in their recovery journey. You learned various tools that you and your loved one can integrate into their recovery plan. In the next chapter, we will discuss in more detail how to work effectively with your loved one in this journey.

CHAPTER 3

Working with Your Loved One Effectively in Recovery

Working effectively with your loved one on their recovery journey requires effort and a shift in mindset to better understand their needs and motivations. To begin, we offer a framework to understand where your loved one is in their recovery journey. This understanding will help you engage with your loved one constructively based on their specific situation and mindset. The rest of the chapter outlines strategies and tools to facilitate collaboration, promote positive changes, and address common challenges so you can reach recovery working together.

The Stages of Change

Recovery requires change. Below we offer and expand on the Stages of Change framework created by the scholars Prochaska and DiClemente (1982). It can help you understand where your loved one is in their recovery and determine how best to help them at each stage. While this model may suggest a step-by-step process, recovery is not linear and is prone to setbacks along the way.

Precontemplation

Your loved one shows no desire to change and is not pursuing treatment. The reason for their inaction may be that they feel stuck, demoralized, dependent, or overwhelmed by a sense of disability.

Arguing with, berating, scaring, threatening, or confronting your loved one may increase their resistance and undermine your efforts. Try to learn why your loved may be resistant to change. Use empathy to strengthen your relationship and build trust so they feel comfortable sharing what is holding them back.

Contemplation

Your loved one recognizes there's a problem and is considering positive behavior changes. But they are unsure if they will be successful and are ambivalent about acting.

Recognize that change is hard but tap into renewed signs of hope they may express. Try to engage your loved one in a discussion of the pros and cons of seeking treatment.

Preparation

Your loved one is ready and planning to make a change soon. They have reached a decisive point to take back their life and independence. But they are still figuring out how to implement behavioral changes.

You can help your loved one develop a plan using the following steps:

- Confirm their expectations for treatment and recovery

- Discuss openly if these expectations are reasonable and achievable

- Identify potential challenges through the treatment process and develop solutions together

- Help your loved one identify and coordinate a larger support network

- Help your loved one refine their treatment plan—it helps to formalize the plan in writing

Behavior Change

Your loved one has started making positive behavior changes and actively engaging in their treatment. They have moved from dependence on you and others to increased self-reliance and determination. However, your loved one may be vulnerable to frustrations and setbacks.

You can help them build and maintain momentum using the following tips:

- Recognize the steps they have taken and reinforce the positive impact they are having

- When setbacks arise, or you sense your loved one becoming discouraged, emphasize the investment they've already made in behavior changes; highlight the gains that they've already made and proven ability to progress; and work with them to develop coping strategies they can use for when setbacks and triggers arise

Maintenance

Your loved has reached recovery. They have accomplished treatment goals and are making continued progress. They have established a healthy routine and overcome many of the challenges to adhere to their treatment plan. They are making efforts to integrate with their community and achieve employment goals.

You can help your loved one maintain this positive momentum by:

- Recognizing and praising their healthier lifestyle, determination, and resolve

- Discussing techniques and approaches that your loved one can employ to avoid reverting to unhealthy behaviors

- Working together to create a plan in case of a relapse

- Reviewing and encouraging new long-term goals, which may evolve over time as your loved achieve new successes

Relapse

Your loved one is likely to experience a recurrence of unhealthy behavior or other setbacks. It is important to help them re-engage quickly and constructively with the treatment process. Use the following strategies:

- Help your loved one understand that relapse is common. Help them problem solve and learn from the relapse. Encourage them to view recovery as a journey.

- Encourage your loved one during this challenging period. Highlight the progress they have made. Help them see the relapse as a temporary setback.

- Assess potential adjustments to the treatment approach and support systems that might prevent future relapses.

- Help your loved one problem solve and learn from the relapse.

- Address any damage to your loved one's self-worth and determination.

EXERCISE: Assessing Your Loved One's Situation

Make a list of the behaviors that may be holding your loved one back. These may include both actions they're taking and actions they're not taking. See if you can understand why your loved one engages in the behavior: for example, "I think you're comfortable staying with the familiar, even if it's not working so well." This is also a useful empathy exercise to gauge how well you understand ambivalence your loved one might be feeling.

When your loved one is open to it, share your observations. Ask whether your assessment of what they might be feeling is correct and which behaviors they would like to change. Be open to the response they offer you, whatever that might be; they're the authority on their own experience. Next, ask if they would like your help pursuing any of the changes the two of you will have identified, so you can focus your own efforts, and respect their wishes, whatever those wishes might be.

Rules for Collaboration

You and your loved one can achieve better outcomes if you work together. The following rules can help you work successfully with your loved one through collaborative decision-making. The goal is to develop treatment and self-care objectives, responsibilities, and action plans together. Practicing these principles can make your loved one, you, and all the people in your support network feel better about the treatment process, because everyone will have a say in it.

You will need to tailor this framework for your specific situation and support network members. Ideally, you and your loved one will review and adapt these principles, with potential input from a healthcare provider. As a caregiver, you might have to initiate the process by drafting principles on your own to share with your loved one. This initiative may also be a sign of your good-faith commitment to work collaboratively. Finally, treatment and self-care approaches should be flexible and adaptable. You may need to revisit yours as your loved one's mental illness and relationships evolve.

Rule 1: *Acceptance*

Many caregivers mistakenly believe that the only path to improvement is for their loved one to change. As a caregiver, it is important for you to recognize that you cannot force your loved one to change things they may not want to change. It is generally more constructive to focus on acceptance. Acceptance means allowing your loved one to be who they are, regardless of whether you agree with them. It is important to recognize and differentiate things that are changeable (such as poor medication adherence or refusal to abstain from street drugs) from those that may be beyond voluntary control and require radical acceptance (such as tolerating negative emotions when they are).

Remember that there are aspects you can change even when your loved one does not change. You have the power to change your reaction to your loved one. You choose how you manage the parts of your loved one that you cannot change. This includes your beliefs about their capabilities, your expectations for them, and the way you approach conversations and express yourself to them.

It is also important not to overly protect your loved one. Sometimes caregivers do everything they can to convince their loved one to accept treatment without success. In these cases, provided there is no danger to them, you may have to let your loved one experience the natural consequences of an untreated illness to persuade them to get treatment.

Sometimes the best lessons in dealing with mental illness are learned from mistakes and failures.

Importantly, acceptance does not mean tolerating behaviors that negatively impact you and your family. Self-destructive behaviors, such as deliberate self-injury or illicit substance use, cannot be ignored, nor can endangering the welfare of minor children. Abusive behavior— physical, emotional, or verbal—is never acceptable. Understanding the different types of abuse can help address unhealthy relationship dynamics. We can then take the necessary actions to remove ourselves from abusive situations, which may involve seeking support from friends and family in a position to help.

Rule 2: *See the Person*

Often, when a loved one falls ill, caregivers tend to shift their focus solely onto the illness and disregard their loved one's personhood. Every conversation revolves around the illness itself, which can make your loved one feel reduced to their condition.

Adopting person-first language can help. Person-first language requires avoiding words that perpetuate stigma and terms that reduce individuals to their symptoms, illnesses, or conditions. For example, instead of saying your loved one "is bipolar" or "is schizophrenic," you would say "They are living with bipolar disorder" or "They have schizophrenia." Research shows that using person-first language positively impacts health outcomes and recovery. When you use person-first language, you actively support your loved one's healing, progress, and personal goals.

Rule 3: *Your Loved One Has Autonomy*

Autonomy is having control and the freedom to make choices in one's life as a unique and independent individual. It is crucial to respect and support your loved one's autonomy in their daily life. Encourage and help them to continue with routine yet essential tasks, such as shopping, recreational activities, and social interactions, to the extent they are capable. A perceived lack of control can lead to increased anxiety, stress, depression, or pessimism for them. Additionally, when your loved one feels that they are the driving force behind their actions, they will be more motivated to pursue change and recovery. Respecting your loved one's autonomy in both small and significant aspects of life helps preserve their dignity, which can be a boost in the recovery journey.

Rule 4: *Supporters Can Help*

Your loved one can achieve better outcomes if they accept support and if supporters participate constructively in their care.

However, beware of helicoptering. Helicoptering occurs when a loved one might feel you're constantly "hovering over" them to control, correct, or admonish their behavior. This persistent monitoring can feel suffocating, disempowering, discouraging, and even angering. Your intentions may well be good but helicoptering often leads the loved one to withdraw and isolate themself.

Rule 5: *Supporters, Loved Ones, and Healthcare Providers Must Collaborate and Communicate*

No one is to blame for the illness. We all work together to achieve recovery. And to do so effectively, we should all communicate what's most important to us to avoid misunderstanding. Good communication is essential for collaboration. Practice empathy, compassion, and respect in conversations. Without good communication, it will be extremely difficult for you to help your loved one. (We talk more about communication in chapter 8, Talking About Mental Illness.) Your loved one may be more willing to do what you suggest if you explain nonjudgmentally why you think it's important. Likewise, you may be more willing to support your loved one's actions if you know their reasons.

Rule 6: *Create an Amicable Family Environment and Show Compassion for Mistakes*

As a caregiver, do your best to create and maintain an amicable, supportive family environment.

Being supportive will help your loved one collaborate in treatment and self-care. Although it may be difficult, try to follow these caregiver dos and don'ts.

Do	Don't
Accept	Argue
Affirm	Blame
Build confidence	Control/Overwhelm
Empathize	Criticize
Be honest	Discriminate
Respect	Dismiss
Be sensitive	Disrespect
Trust	Gaslight
Validate feelings	Infantilize
	Judge
	Provoke
	Punish
	Rebut
	Shame
	Stigmatize

It's especially important to use positive, supportive strategies in the face of mistakes. People with mental illness frequently dwell on their past mistakes and regrettable behaviors during an episode. If you notice that your loved one is actively trying to improve their behavior, you may want to avoid bringing up these prior incidents.

This advice is particularly relevant for people with bipolar disorder. During a hypomanic episode, your loved one may have acted in a reckless and erratic manner, without considering the consequences for themself or their family in the moment. When they regain stability, they often experience deep regret, shame, and embarrassment for their actions. Likewise, during severe depressive episodes, a person may disengage from their role as a worker, student, or homemaker or otherwise cease to participate in activities through no "fault" of their own.

If you, as a caregiver, find yourself feeling hurt and awaiting an apology from your loved one for past events, try to recognize if their behavior was a consequence of their illness. It can be helpful for you to develop a tough outer skin and not necessarily take things personally if your loved one says or does things that may feel hurtful. Be aware that your loved one may be loath to discuss painful past experiences not out of disregard for you but because of their own embarrassment or shame. Acknowledge to your loved one how painful or upsetting it may be for them to think back on the consequences of a past episode. Express regret for the episode, rather than for what they did. Blame the illness not the person. This approach is not only comforting but can help your loved one become more open and engage with their support team if their condition worsens. You might also find therapy or some other means to process your own complex feelings, independently of your loved one.

Specific examples of these types of communications are discussed further in chapter 8, Talking About Mental Illness.

Rule 7: *Approach Emotions and Arguments Thoughtfully and De-escalate When Possible*

It's impossible to contain all emotions and avoid all arguments. Agitation is a common symptom of SMIs. Understand triggers for anger and be prepared to address them constructively. Your loved one's anger may be triggered by external, internal, traumatic, and symptom triggers. It can also occur spontaneously for no apparent reason at all. Should you bear the brunt of a loved one's anger, you may sometimes feel inclined to question whether your loved one's anger is "justified"; it may be more productive instead to acknowledge that he or she feels angry, and empathize with their sense of distress and discord.

You should expect and accept reasonable expressions of emotions from your loved one. But you should try to identify their cause and work thoughtfully to address them at the root. The active listening techniques we'll discuss in chapter 8 may help you understand the causes of your loved one's anger when it arises. Bear in mind that if your loved one can't express their anger constructively, it may escalate. Your loved one may demonstrate physical agitation; it may even become a potential emergency.

Tense situations will likely arise throughout your loved one's recovery journey. It is prudent to learn de-escalation techniques that can defuse these types of situations, such as:

- Find a private space. It may help to move your loved one away from public areas and into a private space for conversations, and to ensure privacy from other family members, including children.

- Institute a cooling-off period. Know when to propose a cooling-off period, particularly when processing highly emotionally charged material. Also be prepared to postpone discussions that may become heated.

- Show empathy and avoid judgment. Focus on understanding your loved one's emotions. Whether or not you believe their feelings are justified, they are real to them. Convey that they are not alone, and many others have similar feelings.

- Respect personal boundaries. Maintaining some distance from your loved one to allow personal space can reduce anxiety and prevent outbursts. Don't block them from leaving the room if they need to.

- Avoid excessive reactions. Stay calm and rational. How you respond to your loved one's behavior can determine whether the situation escalates or diffuses. Validate their emotions while addressing inappropriate behavior.

- Disregard challenging questions. Engaging with challenging questions often leads to power struggles. Redirect your loved one's attention to the matter at hand.

- Establish boundaries. If your loved one is confrontational, defensive, or disruptive, provide clear, concise, and enforceable limits. Offer respectful choices and consequences. Suggest options and flexibility to avoid unnecessary conflict.

- Allow moments of silence. By allowing silence, you provide an opportunity for the person to reflect on the situation and determine their next steps.

- Allow time for decision-making. When someone is upset, their ability to think clearly may be impaired. Give them time to process the situation and any information you have shared.

- Stay safe. Productive discussions cannot occur if all parties do not feel safe. If either you or your loved one is concerned about your physical safety, you should say so and not allow a heated discussion to continue unless and until you both feel physically safe.

Again, chapter 8, Talking About Mental Illness, offers more strategies.

Rule 8: *Loved One Has Self-Determination and Ownership over Their Treatment*

Self-determined people proactively work toward specific goals and initiate change in their lives, rather than relying on others to dictate or act on their behalf. Their actions are guided by personal preferences and interests. They advocate for themselves, actively participate in problem-solving, and engage in decision-making processes regarding their lives. It is important to note that self-determination does not mean handling everything independently; rather, it involves taking actions that lead to positive changes and improvements in one's life.

Your loved one must have ownership of their treatment, which means:

- Feeling a sense of autonomy and control over decisions about their treatment

- Appreciating that they have ultimate responsibility for their treatment and self-care

You can help your loved one exercise self-determination in many ways. To embrace self-determination, they must possess the ability to set goals, assess various options, make choices, and then exert effort to accomplish those goals. You can encourage and assist your loved one to execute on each of these components.

You should defer to your loved one's preferences and objectives unless their judgment has been substantially impaired. This control will make your loved one more likely to continue treatment, engage in self-care, and agree to family participation in their activities. No one likes to have their decisions made for them.

Rule 9: *Encourage Self-Empowerment and Practice Shared Decision-Making in Treatment*

Those of us with mental health challenges often feel powerless and out of control in our own lives. So, we may rely heavily on our caregivers to make treatment decisions, either due to difficulty accepting diagnoses or uncertainty about our own choices. Sometimes, a loved one may adopt an indifferent or passive role in their treatment decisions, making their caregiver the de facto decision maker; that dynamic can be at odds with self-empowerment. As the caregiver of a person living with SMI, you'll need to work to encourage your loved one's self-empowerment, and to respect it. It's pivotal in their journey toward recovery.

One way to do this is to consistently engage your loved one in open-ended discussions about their treatment and their experience of living with their symptoms. This approach can allow them to express their desires and take ownership of their mental illness and treatment. Work to respect and trust their decisions. This may allow your loved one to feel more liberated and significantly improve the relationship dynamic.

In chapter 5, Navigating Psychiatric Treatment, we will explore a shared decision-making approach. Shared decision-making can encourage people with mental illness to take ownership and responsibility for their care. In this approach, a patient clearly communicates their priorities to their caregiver and healthcare providers, and together they establish a treatment plan. This strategy focuses on helping people living with SMI pursue their life goals—personal recovery—rather than solely addressing symptoms and side effects. It proves highly effective in treatment and self-empowerment. Healthcare providers should share their expertise on available treatment options and advise if your loved one is considering options that are risky or unlikely to be effective. Your loved one should ultimately decide. You can offer your help but must respect their decision.

Rule 10: *Plan Ahead*

You, your loved one, and all members of your support team should recognize that SMI may sometimes impair your loved one's ability to exercise reasonable judgment about treatment decisions. Discuss and agree on an action plan in the event of an emergency, including the potential need for involuntary treatment. Chapter 5 discusses planning for emergencies in more detail.

Rule 11: *Have a Clear Objective for Care*

The illness—its symptoms and effects on your loved one's quality of life—is the object of the care your loved one receives. Treatment should be recovery oriented, person centered, and wellness targeted. Family conflicts or stresses are treated separately, if necessary. Family therapy, which focuses on interactions between its members, may be relevant when there are concerns about negative or disruptive communication styles (see the table of dos and don'ts above).

Rule 12: *Use Evidence-Based Education and Resources*

Loved ones and caregivers benefit when they are informed about mental illness and have access to appropriate resources. Rely on trustworthy resources, including credentialed and knowledgeable healthcare providers, to learn about evidence-based and emerging best practices. Rely on scientific principles and support to make informed treatment decisions. You can find a list of reliable resources at the end of this book.

Rule 13: *Seek Ongoing Guidance and Skills Training*

The healthcare providers you work with should provide you and your loved one with ongoing guidance and skills training, especially for crisis management. This enables you and your support team to better manage the illness.

Rule 14: *Recognize the Limitations Illness Can Cause*

One pitfall is failing to recognize that your loved one's actions are often a result of their illness, not intentional behavior or a character flaw. To help identify these misperceptions and improve understanding, try the following exercise. List your loved one's unhealthy behaviors and categorize them as controllable or beyond their control; have your loved one do the same. Each of you can then comment on missing or misclassified items from the other's list. For example, you may think that your loved one sleeps late because they are lazy or unmotivated, but they may be over-medicated, depressed, or both.

You may need to work with your loved one to modify their pursuits or life goals based on the limitations that the illness might impose. Help your loved one cope with these changes by promoting adaptability and practicing compassion.

Rule 15: *Use a Problem-Solving Approach*

Use a problem-solving approach to help you, your loved one, and healthcare providers address issues together. Try breaking down complicated issues into small, manageable steps that are more easily addressed.

EXERCISE: Considering Your Current Relationship

As a caregiver, you play a critical role in motivating your loved one to make positive changes. Your loved one is more likely to collaborate when they feel you care about their specific goals. This care requires understanding what's important to your loved one and their motivations. Try the following exercise to gauge your understanding of your loved one's goals and priorities:

1. Write down three short-term goals and three long-term goals you believe your loved one has for their recovery (keep in mind that goals should be S.M.A.R.T., as discussed in chapters 1 and 7).

2. Ask your loved one to write down three short-term goals and three long-term goals they have for their recovery.

3. Share your lists with each other.

4. After reviewing the lists, compare them and discuss the differences between your loved one's stated goals and your understanding of their goals.

5. Work together to agree on a single list of three short-term and three long-term goals for your loved one's recovery.

By completing this exercise, you and your loved one will develop and refine a shared understanding of your loved one's goals. The better you understand your loved one's goals, the better positioned you are to help in their recovery.

Conclusion

In conclusion, working effectively with your loved one in their recovery journey requires patience, understanding, and a willingness to adapt. By recognizing your loved one's situation, following key rules to collaborate effectively, and utilizing strategies to promote positive changes and address common challenges, you can provide invaluable support to your loved one. Recovery is not always a linear process, and setbacks may occur along the way—but with your support and guidance, your loved one can navigate these challenges and move toward a healthier, fulfilling life.

Supporting Your Loved One on the Treatment Journey

CHAPTER 4

Caregivers and other stakeholders may sometimes misinterpret, fail to comprehend, or otherwise have misperceptions about the nature of SMI. The resulting misunderstandings can further drive stigma and strain relationships, hindering your loved one's ability to act in their own best interests. Learning and understanding the truth about SMI—its manageability and the potential for a fulfilling life in recovery—can counteract its debilitating effects.

As isolated as you might feel, countless people have gone through similar experiences. We write this having gone through them too. The recovery journey will bring challenges—such as differing views on treatment, issues with control, and changes in your relationship—and these challenges can be overcome through empathy, compassion, understanding, acceptance, honesty, and respect.

In this chapter, we'll offer you skills to ease the tensions that stigma and the experience of SMI have likely caused in your relationship with your loved one, so you can strengthen that relationship.

Approaching Your Loved One with Honesty and Openness

Your relationship with your loved one may be fraught with misunderstanding and miscommunication. And you're both bound to say the wrong thing sometimes. Reframing the dialogue can dramatically improve the results. Seemingly subtle shifts in tone, from demanding "You have to stop" and "Listen to me" to asking "Can I help?" and "Would you like my opinion?", can profoundly improve your relationship. Always remember that the first instinct of a person with SMI, when their relationships deteriorate, is to isolate and withdraw, which will break down communication. It is critical to maintain that communication instead.

You may desperately try to protect your loved one from the pain and suffering that is part of any SMI. It's a natural impulse when any human sees someone they love suffering. You may also try to protect yourself or other members of the family from the possible consequences of the illness. Maybe you try to control the uncontrollable—and feel like you're looking for comfort and safety where there is none. We all sometimes try to control the uncontrollable by looking for security and predictability. But we can never avoid uncertainty. Not knowing is what makes us afraid—and is part of the journey. There can be fleeting moments of reprieve, too. And there must always be hope.

Helping Your Loved One While Preserving Your Relationship

Here, we'll consider common experiences that can create significant conflict with your loved one and potential strategies to address them. They may help you reduce and manage uncertainty. That said, it's important to avoid overstating your knowledge or understanding of your loved one's condition and situation when engaging with them. It's generally safer to approach discussions with openness and interest in hearing from your loved one what they're experiencing, to explore if they would like your help.

Your loved one refuses to get help. Your approach needs to be balanced. If your loved one tells you they're not sick, refrain from threats or coercion to get treatment. Keep the conversation nonantagonistic by listening to them. Try discussing triggers of mental illness and symptoms that your loved one may be experiencing—like stress, sleep disruptions, or drugs and alcohol use—if they resist the suggestion that they may be experiencing mental illness. For example, you could say "I notice you haven't been sleeping as much lately" or "You seem to be under a lot more stress lately, perhaps that's impacting how you feel day-to-day?" This approach can help normalize mental illness and take a step toward discussing it. Still, caregivers can seek strategies in order to not stand by idly when they observe symptoms that their loved one may not notice. It can prove valuable to anticipate situations such as these, and develop preferred action plans, before they arrive. For example, "If there should come a time when I think you are having symptoms but you may not agree, I'd like your permission in advance to communicate my concerns to the clinician treating you."

Your loved one refuses to accept a diagnosis. People with mental illness often experience shock or denial, sometimes both, when they receive a diagnosis. It may not come as a surprise to you, the caregiver, and you may even feel relieved that there is finally a diagnosis. But there are many reasons that your loved one may resist the diagnosis, including the stigma it brings, lack of information about the diagnosis, and lack of insight into their own behavior, often a symptom of SMI.

It nearly always helps for a caregiver to validate these feelings, whether or not your loved one makes that need obvious. It is also important to determine what your loved one even understands about the diagnosis. They may have misconceptions or wrong information based on stigma or their own past experiences. You can assemble educational materials and offer them to your loved one in part to highlight the prevalence of mental illness.

Your loved one reluctantly accepts a diagnosis but does not consistently do what's best for them. It may help to remind your loved one that they can live the life that they had before they got sick, once they've learned to adapt to and deal with their symptoms, and that treatment works. It can also help to show them examples of people living well with mental illness. However, it is best not to say you understand a particular experience unless you do.

Self-sabotage, like deliberately not taking care of themselves, or disavowal of treatment are common for people dealing with SMI. Peers can be a tremendous source of inspiration, particularly when your loved one is dealing with something you don't understand. Your loved one should always decide if they would like to engage with their peers. Allowing them to come to this conclusion on their own may facilitate acceptance of their diagnosis.

Your loved one accepts their diagnosis but is not adhering to medical treatment. You may want to try to enforce your loved one's adherence with their medical treatment, particularly taking their medication as prescribed. Rather than try to control or supervise their behavior, it may be more constructive to ask your loved one what makes them reluctant to accept treatment. You can ask them if they would like your help researching medications or speaking with their psychiatrist. You should also encourage them to get more information from their doctor. For instance, if the reason they refuse to take medication is its side effects, encourage them to talk to their psychiatrist about managing these side effects. Doing this empowers your loved one with agency. Many common side effects—such as weight gain, drowsiness, sexual dysfunction, or movement problems—can be effectively managed through a variety of strategies that your loved one may not realize exist. In addition, you can offer to join them in speaking with their psychiatrist if your support would be helpful.

You need to recognize that your loved one's treatment is their personal choice. You may need to allow your loved one to face the risks of not adhering to medical treatment. You might acknowledge that you respect their free will not to seek treatment while making them aware of the risks they are accepting.

Your loved one does the minimum and doesn't seem fully committed to recovery. You can always gently encourage your loved one to do more, but never forcefully. It can be tremendously positive to remind your loved one of past dreams and new ambitions. You should reinforce dreams that remain achievable while recognizing the new constraints mental illness may impose. You can also ask your loved one what they would like to do if they were well. This might include returning to school or getting a job. And, once your loved one has some goals or visions elaborated, you can help them achieve those goals by assembling informational materials. You can speak to the loved one about what they found or place material in a convenient spot where the loved one can access it on their own.

Your loved one is highly negative. First and foremost, never argue. It can be very difficult to experience your loved one's negativity, particularly if it's directed at you. But if you don't take your loved one's feelings as they are and endeavor to truly understand them, you'll never be able to move forward. Avoid statements like "Everything is okay" or "There's no reason to be down," which may be counterproductive as they fail to recognize the reality of the illness and what your loved one is experiencing. Instead, accept and recognize how your loved one is feeling—try to say things like "I know that you are feeling down" and "If you want to talk about it, I'm here"—and do your best to help your loved one work through it. Always offer to talk; never say "We have to talk." It can help to remind your loved one of past times when they overcame a struggle.

Finally, be aware of the resources that you may need, as a caregiver, to keep yourself going when things get tough. It can be very hard to be the one to maintain hope when your loved one is struggling. Speaking to a friend or a therapist can help you give yourself the energy you need to persist and keep resentment, impatience, and other emotions from filtering into your conversations with your loved one.

Your loved one sabotages their recovery. Many people with mental illness are afraid of failure and disappointment. They may think it's inevitable. They may fear relapse. Some people with SMIs may feel that they don't deserve to feel better. As a result, they may unwittingly or deliberately commit acts of self-sabotage, even when they're doing well. You should reinforce to your loved one that they can achieve and live a fulfilling life. Don't take sabotage as a permanent break from recovery. Take it as an expression of how your loved one is feeling, and communicate openly with them to help them process these feelings.

Your loved one has a setback. If your loved one experiences a setback, you may be tempted to question whether they somehow caused it. Did they stop their medicines? Did they fail to recognize symptoms that could impact their judgment? It can be hard to balance such concerns with maintaining empathy.

Acknowledge the disappointment. You can also try to put the situation in better context or reframe it. For example, it may help to applaud striving, willingness to take a risk, and anything your loved one might have learned from a setback or disappointment. It can help to remind your loved one of past challenges they overcame.

The recovery journey is not easy. It can be full of twists and turns. So, you should try to be adaptable and flexible. It's also important not to think that because your loved one was able to do something on an earlier day, they can do the same thing today. Each day will be different, and it can be difficult and take a while to get into a consistent positive routine.

You repeatedly push your loved one to act. You should never nag your loved one when they refuse to act, as this may backfire. Instead of doing what is asked, your loved one may isolate and withdraw, and if you nag, they may entrench further in isolation.

It is often more productive to ask your loved one, nonjudgmentally and with genuine curiosity, what they think is holding them back and if they would like help. Never dismiss their reasons for failing to act—empathize and work with them to determine how to move forward.

Your loved one is having a hard time with a specific obstacle. Recognize the challenges that your loved one faces, even if you can't understand why something is difficult for them. You cannot will your loved one into action. They must have the will. So, instead of pushing when your loved one is having a hard time, focus on motivating and engaging with your loved one so that their desire to act comes from within. It is important not to ignore your loved one's challenges when you do this. Focus on understanding the challenges and try to help your loved one overcome them, on their terms.

Your loved one withdraws and isolates. This can be one of the most heartbreaking situations a caregiver can experience. Your loved one may refuse to engage at all. They may refuse to leave their room. One of the best approaches you can take in these moments is to offer help, even as you leave your loved one space to ensure they don't feel crowded or pressured, particularly when what they're going through is likely painful. Check in on your loved one from time to time and ask them if you can help. You can offer to lend an ear, or sometimes it helps merely to be a supportive presence who needs not say anything but will just be there. You can bring snacks and meals into the room.

If you are genuinely concerned that your loved one's withdrawal and isolation reflect the severity of undertreated symptoms, tell them so with compassion and honesty. Offer to make an appointment with their psychiatrist if they have not seen them in a while. But be careful not to make the loved one feel like a burden. An emotional support animal can often greatly help the loved one manage their loneliness.

You and your loved one disagree on important actions. Disagreements on important actions, such as treatment adherence, are common. When there's a disagreement between you and your loved one, you can express concern. You can try to reach an agreement with your loved one and partner with them to help achieve the desired outcome. In specific circumstances, you can suggest speaking with your loved one to try to agree on certain actions, like how best to react in a crisis, in advance. As you will read below, planning for this crisis can help bring order to an otherwise chaotic situation.

Your loved one may be unwilling to cooperate because they don't believe a crisis will occur. Even so, giving them a sense of control and ownership over their condition in advance may help overcome this reluctance. It will help reduce the potential uncertainty in a crisis because they will have a plan for what to do if they have difficulty exercising judgment during an episode.

Your loved one is in a crisis moment. When your loved one is in crisis, they may not be able to exercise sound judgment. They might be highly manic or deeply depressed, or they could simply be experiencing an enormous amount of distress. They may deny that they are in a crisis altogether. They may want to be left alone. You may feel like telling them what to do, for their own good. But they can't be told what to do.

These moments will be very tough. It can be very hard to see your loved one in pain or behaving in ways that seem to risk their safety. Be careful not to push your loved one away. Offer to listen to whatever it is they're feeling or what might be concerning them. Ask if you can help in any way. If you previously agreed on a plan of action in a crisis, it is time to execute that plan. If your loved one has a psychiatric advance directive (see chapter 5, Navigating Psychiatric Treatment) it can provide a roadmap. Remind them that they planned for this situation. Remain as calm as you can under the circumstances. Your energy and anxiety may contribute to your loved one's mood. You might ask your loved one if they would like to speak or see their doctor.

If your loved one has hurt themself or others, or is talking about hurting themself or others, they may need to get professional treatment as soon as possible, whether voluntarily or involuntarily. Confirm they do not have access to any unsecure weapons or other means of harm. You may have to make the decision for them to get the urgent help they need.

Negotiating Relationships with Healthcare Providers

If there's disagreement on healthcare providers, work together. You must always remember that it is your loved one who will have the relationship with any healthcare providers you work with and that they must be comfortable with their selection. If your loved one expresses reservations about a provider, take these concerns seriously. It is also important to recognize that healthcare professionals can also harbor their own biases, may not know enough about a certain condition, or may not be the right personality fit, which may compromise your loved one's treatment. For example, a psychiatrist may prematurely or abruptly provide a negative prognosis that leaves your loved one feeling demoralized. Or they may deliver their opinions insensitively.

In such cases, there are certainly times it can be useful to find a different psychiatrist or other professional better suited to treating your loved one. It might be helpful to seek clarification from the provider or consider seeking a second opinion. This additional effort and selectivity can help your loved one better come to terms with their ultimate diagnosis and treatment plan. It is also very valuable because your loved one may ultimately invest significant time and energy into their relationship with a psychiatrist. You and they will want to make the right choice for pursuing a longer-term relationship and treatment approach.

Barring emergencies, you should not speak separately to your loved one's healthcare provider without your loved one's prior consent. Unless there's an emergency, always obtain your loved one's consent before discussing their treatment with healthcare providers. Respect their privacy and autonomy in managing their healthcare. Inform your loved one before reaching out to their provider and invite them to participate in the conversation. Promote open communication among all parties involved to foster collaboration and empower your loved one in their treatment decisions. A healthcare provider, in turn, needs your loved one's explicit consent to discuss their condition or treatment with any third party, including caregivers.

Of course, where fundamental issues of safety and self-care arise, maintaining your loved one's privacy and minimizing your input into their treatment may not always be feasible. But if you respect your loved one's right to own their treatment and recovery, and work to put them in control of what happens with their providers as often as possible, you'll help build trust between yourself, your loved one, and their providers.

Be careful not to appear as though you're siding with a healthcare provider against your loved one. Avoid appearing to side with healthcare providers against your loved one's wishes. Evaluate your motives carefully if you feel compelled to advocate for more aggressive care or support a provider's recommendation that your loved one opposes. Colluding with providers without your loved one's knowledge can damage trust and strain your relationship. Instead, engage in open dialogue with your loved one to address disagreements and explore mutually acceptable solutions.

If you feel there's a problem that needs resolution urgently, and your loved one seems to disagree or doesn't seem as motivated to solve that problem, consider the previous section's guidance on what to do when your loved one is having a hard time with an obstacle.

Helping Your Loved One Preserve Their Control

Do not try to "fix" a situation, or your loved one. Caregivers often think they can fix a situation or a person. The truth is that in many situations, you can help, and your loved one can help themselves, but you cannot "fix" someone with SMI. You must accept that, to limit your own disappointment and frustration.

It can be hard to accept the things you cannot change. It's often useful for you, as a caregiver, to obtain your own mental health treatment—to talk to a therapist or other professional on a regular basis.

Do not take control of decisions. Let your loved one take control; offer them support as they may need it. Try not to take control of decisions unless your loved one is willing to accept this. And even then, respect your loved one's desires and autonomy as much as you can. It's incredibly hurtful to feel disempowered and without control over one's life. Any action taken during a crisis—especially involuntary hospitalization—must be very carefully considered; it may leave your loved one feeling disrespected, or even violated, and it may make them reluctant to trust you or their providers in the future.

Your loved one is ultimately in control of their recovery and life. It's important to defer to them whenever possible and offer to help them exercise their control. Never try to force action.

Of course, sometimes you may need to exercise "tough love," or make clear to your loved one that a situation they're in is likely to be unsustainable and change of some kind will need to happen. These situations may include illicit drug use, criminal activity, or other potentially destructive behavior than may be harmful to your loved one or others. In such moments, it's crucial not to punish your loved one. Your task is to make it clear to them, in a kind and loving way, what you see going on and what you would like to see change—recognizing and validating what they must be feeling or the feelings that may accompany thoughts of change. You could approach your loved one about this potentially delicate situation by saying something like "I know that your situation may be difficult to control, but it's important to address for your treatment to be more effective." Tactically, this might mean making certain resources or "rewards" (such as money or housing) contingent on their willingness to abide by ground rules as discussed in the Wellness Plan chapter.

Do not threaten punitive actions. You may be tempted to punish your loved one for lack of action, which can backfire and aggravate the situation. Of course, you should take action to discourage harmful behavior such as substance use and self-harm—but these actions shouldn't be meted out to punish. Instead, set limits or boundaries—like limiting access to financial resources—as kindly yet firmly as you can. Keep in mind that such actions may be met with anger on your loved one's part. Be cautious about making statements that sound like ultimatums. For example, instead of saying something like "Either stop drinking or leave my house," which can sound like a threat of punishment, consider "You cannot continue to live here if you continue to drink." Be prepared to enforce consequences if you set limits or create disincentives.

Deal with rude and disrespectful behavior in as balanced and kind a way as possible. A person with mental illness may at times be rude and disrespectful. Sometimes they're angry at their illness and may project their anger onto you, telling you things like "It's all your fault."

It can be hard for each of you to recognize each other's distress. It is important to remind yourselves that such moments are often the illness talking.

You may have a difficult time separating your loved one from their illness. But acting out, which is easy to personalize, is often a projection of emotions your loved one may feel toward themself or their illness, propelled by the disempowerment many feel when they become ill and others come to control their treatment and life.

And of course, seek care for yourself so you can process your own feelings and avoid burning out. Being a caregiver can be hard. Taking care of yourself will help you build the resilience you need.

Set boundaries for yourself with your loved one. You'll encounter complex situations as a caregiver; your loved one may struggle with feeling like a burden, disappointment, or source of stress to you. Respond with care for their well-being and respect for their agency. Seek permission before taking any action. Ask your loved one if they need help, when they're struggling, and how they'd like to be helped, or if they'd like your opinion. Sometimes, the best reaction is to back off and be patient. Most importantly, always act with empathy and compassion. Make sure your loved one feels loved and needed.

Consider involuntary hospitalization only as last resort. An involuntary hospitalization should always be the last course of action. It may be unavoidable, if your loved one is greatly impaired. It can also be very traumatizing, for your loved one and you. Your loved one may resent you for it, becoming reluctant to share how they're really feeling with you, even if their condition deteriorates. A voluntary hospitalization is nearly always the best option—except when involuntary hospitalization is needed to protect the safety of your loved one or others.

Conclusion

This chapter offered strategies for you to help your loved one withstand and overcome the challenges of SMI. You also learned ways to address common difficulties you may encounter, from treatment reluctance to setbacks and crises. Preserving your loved one's autonomy—avoiding impulses to control or "fix" them—is paramount. At the same time, you must be able and prepared to act in moments of heightened risk to your loved one and provide input on treatment—within boundaries you and your loved one agree on. The chapter underscores the need for open communication and collaboration between you, your loved one, healthcare providers, and your support team—and crucially, maintaining empathy, understanding, and hope for your loved one.

CHAPTER 5

Navigating Psychiatric Treatment

Psychiatric treatment is vital to caring for a loved one with SMI. And your involvement in your loved one's treatment is vital. This chapter guides you through the complexities of psychiatric treatment, empowering you to play an active, informed role in your loved one's well-being. You'll learn more about mental health conditions, treatment stages, finding the right psychiatrist, and handling emergencies. Ultimately, the way in which you participate in your loved one's care depends on their wishes.

In the Beginning

Being well-informed is essential to receiving effective psychiatric treatment. Knowledge of common conditions and their symptoms can help you recognize early warning signs and seek help sooner. Early intervention can significantly improve outcomes and prevent disruptions to your loved one's life and that of those around them.

Knowing more about mental illness can also empower you and your loved one, reducing uncertainties about conditions and treatments. A basic working knowledge of these topics—as you've begun to build reading this book—can help you navigate future challenges.

It's important to consult reputable sources, like those mentioned in chapter 1, Understanding Your Situation, or the resources section at the end of the book. Also, always talk to healthcare providers about any information you've learned on your own to confirm it. It can also be helpful to take an online screening, such as those from Mental Health America (MHA).

Early Intervention

Knowing when to seek psychiatric care is often difficult, particularly when symptoms first arise. Denial and stigma may create obstacles, and it may take many years to receive a proper diagnosis. Recognizing early the signs of a mental health challenge positions you to act sooner. Research indicates that delays in treatment can lead to more severe outcomes (McLaughlin 2004). Earlier access to treatment and coping strategies can prevent worsening of symptoms, improving your loved one's medical results and quality of life and reducing risks to work, family, school, and lifestyle.

Initial Examination

An initial examination might be conducted by a primary care doctor (PCP), psychiatrist, psychiatric nurse practitioner, social worker, or psychologist. Remember: Not all providers have the expertise to treat SMIs, so it is important to find a provider with this specialization.

Many caregivers will first turn to a PCP. The primary challenge for PCPs is to rule out potential non-psychiatric causes of psychiatric symptoms, like thyroid issues, vitamin deficiencies, or infections like Lyme disease. It's also crucial at this stage to assess substance use, which can significantly impact emotions, thoughts, and behavior. Note, however, that substance use and mental illness often coexist.

PCPs can diagnose and treat mental illnesses like anxiety and depression, referring you to specialists as needed. It's often helpful for your PCP to collaborate with specialist providers to monitor and address any physical health concerns your loved one may have. Life expectancy for people with SMI may be reduced by up to twenty-five years (National Association of State Mental Health Program Directors 2006) due to factors such as weight, metabolic side effects of medications, tobacco dependence, and lack of healthcare access. Your loved one may not always be able to attend to their physical health, so this is an area where you can help.

Psychiatrists

A psychiatrist is a medical doctor who focuses on mental health. They diagnose conditions, prescribe medication, and offer various therapeutic approaches. While there are multiple healthcare providers who can address mental illness, psychiatrists typically undergo the most extensive education and clinical training. Many psychiatrists have specializations, such as child, adolescent, or addiction psychiatry. Due to their comprehensive training, psychiatrists are equipped to handle complex mental health issues that may go beyond the scope of a PCP.

Finding a Psychiatrist

When you are seeking a suitable psychiatrist, speaking to friends or family who also live with mental illness can be a great place to start. You should consider a range of other factors, including cost, convenience, and availability. You can ask your PCP for a recommendation. There are also many online directories that may help find a psychiatrist and/or therapist. Some of the best-known ones include Psychology Today, US News & World Report, and Zencare. Keep in mind that some directories only require a fee to be listed. Nonprofits may also be able to provide referrals to healthcare provider directories for specific communities. *If you have insurance, it typically offers a directory of providers that are in-network.* Some specialties—such as addiction, child, and geriatric psychiatry—also have their own professional guides or organizations.

Carefully evaluate the qualifications and experience of candidates you find. Consider client reviews that may be available—but bear in mind that they may skew to the most positive and negative experiences; avoid putting too much weight on any single review.

You can also consult medical centers often affiliated with medical schools. Check the best medical schools first in the *US News & World Report*. Doctors who work for the affiliated medical center often have a private practice as well. It can also help to research members of industry organizations and nonprofits. Authors who have written about a specific mental health condition in reputable sources may be able to recommend psychiatrists. Academic directories include PubMed and Google Scholar.

Screening Psychiatrists

Once you've identified a doctor or multiple doctors to consider, you must screen them—determine if they really fit your loved one's situation and needs. The following are some important items to keep in mind when screening. You can also find these questions and other free tools online at New Harbinger's website for this book (http://www.newharbinger.com /53837).

Insurance: Do they accept your insurance? It's crucial to know what your benefits cover because you will typically want an ongoing, longer-term relationship with the psychiatrist.

Education: Where did they complete medical school, residency, and post-residency?

Academic affiliation: Do they teach psychiatry? If so, this may reflect a stronger reputation and recognition of their expertise. They may also be more familiar with scientific research—which, if relevant to your condition, may provide them with useful insights for your treatment.

Hospital affiliation: Do they have a hospital affiliation and access to ancillary services such as partial hospital outpatient programs if needed?

Areas of expertise: How relevant is their expertise to you? Do you want a generalist or someone with expertise in a subspecialty?

Publications: Have they published any articles in peer-reviewed journals or books, or produced any videos?

Years of experience: Are you comfortable with their level of experience?

Website: Does their website and description of their practice indicate a good fit for you?

Background: Do they have any disciplinary actions or other issues that concern you? You can search your state medical board for these.

It can be helpful to select a few providers, do some initial screening, and then ask your loved one for their opinion. The final assessment of a healthcare provider should be based on your loved one's goals, values, and preferences. Once you and your loved one have settled on a good candidate, book an initial appointment with them. Then, prepare for that appointment.

Conducting Your Initial Appointment

During the first appointment, be prepared to discuss symptoms, their onset, duration, severity, and potential triggers. Keeping a journal or using an app for monitoring can be helpful. Provide information on past diagnoses, treatments, and medications, including doses, effectiveness, and side effects. It's prudent for you or your loved one to keep a record of medications. Your PCP and pharmacist may provide your medication record.

Good doctors often seek permission to speak with previous clinicians and obtain medical records. A good psychiatrist will also welcome your questions. If they dismiss your concerns, it could indicate they may limit your involvement in care.

Finally, it's empowering for your loved one to approach a potential clinician with their own concerns about treatment. Here are some questions (which you can also find at http://www.newharbinger.com/53837) you can encourage your loved one to ask as applicable:

- What is your treatment approach?

- How can my caregiver be involved in my care?

- How do you balance treatment goals with my life goals?

- How will your treatment plan incorporate my cultural background and beliefs?

- What are my medication options, and what symptoms do they treat?

- What potential side effects should I be aware of?

- How can side effects be managed?

- Are there any interactions with my other medications?

- How do I contact you for medication concerns outside of appointments?

- What is the best way to reach you?

- Can you recommend additional resources?

Medication discussions are essential as they play a significant role in recovery for many with SMI. Nonadherence due to factors such as denial, side effects, perceived lack of efficacy, and lack of family support can lead to relapses. It's crucial to discuss concerns with your provider promptly, as most can be addressed. Set realistic expectations that finding the right medication may take time and experimentation.

Assessing Fit

As a caregiver, attending your loved one's first appointment with their psychiatrist can help with assessing fit. You can express your concerns, ask questions, offer support, and take notes on the discussion. If your loved one is dissatisfied with their experiences with previous psychiatrists, the initial visit with a new provider is a chance to encourage them to share what went wrong.

The primary goal of the first meeting is to evaluate whether your loved one and the psychiatrist are a good match. A strong therapeutic relationship, characterized by warmth, interest, and responsiveness, can significantly impact treatment outcomes.

After several appointments, encourage your loved one to reflect on their connection with the psychiatrist by considering:

Comfort: Did I feel comfortable talking to them?

Empathy: Did I feel they genuinely cared about what matters to me?

Positivity: Did they convey optimism and hope?

Openness: Did I feel free to express my thoughts?

Respect: Did they answer my questions thoughtfully?

Answering no to any of these may suggest the psychiatrist isn't the right fit. Discuss any concerns with your loved one and encourage them to address them with the provider. For your convenience, you can also find these questions online at http://www.newharbinger.com/53837.

Assessing a Provider's Treatment Approach

Treatment should be person-centered and tailored to your loved one's needs, aiming to support their recovery journey. Your loved one should have a say in the services they receive and who's involved in their recovery team. This team will work together to help your loved one achieve both clinical and lifestyle goals.

Shared decision-making is essential in person-centered care. Your loved one, you, their psychiatrist, and others on their support team collaborate to make treatment decisions, considering different perspectives such as the psychiatrist's medical expertise, your loved one's lived experience and goals, and your insights. Importantly, shared decision-making allows a patient to play a direct role in their care, which may make them more likely to adhere to treatment (Fiorillo et al. 2020). This was our experience.

Navigating Diagnosis and Prognosis

Getting a proper diagnosis is key, and only a qualified healthcare provider can offer one. Since there are no simple tests for mental illness, the provider will review your loved one's history and symptoms to make a diagnosis. Still, there are steps you can take to facilitate this process.

Your observations can provide valuable context. Your loved one may not share all their challenges due to stigma, shame, denial, or lack of insight, so your input can fill gaps. Be persistent and patient, because getting an accurate diagnosis can take time and may involve some trial and error.

Keep in mind that reactions to diagnosis can vary—some may struggle with acceptance, while others may feel relief. Supporting your loved one through this process is essential. Ultimately, it's important for your loved one to accept their diagnosis; that's critical for creating and committing to an effective treatment plan. It's also important that this diagnosis be and feel right—one that explains what is happening and makes sense to your loved one and to you. If a diagnosis doesn't seem consistent with symptoms, seeking a second opinion is acceptable.

A hopeful prognosis can motivate recovery. However, providers might offer a cautious outlook. If so, remind your loved one that every journey is unique, and with the right support and treatment, they can pursue a better future.

Treatment Methods Your Provider May Recommend

A combination of medication and psychotherapy often yields the best results in treating SMIs (First 2022). PCPs and psychiatrists may lean toward medication for quick symptom relief, but therapy is just as important for long-term effectiveness. It's crucial to remember that each SMI may require a specific treatment approach. Working with a qualified psychiatrist can help tailor the treatment to your loved one's specific needs.

To shed more light on the treatment of SMIs, we spoke with Joseph Goldberg, a leading SMI psychiatrist. He shared valuable insights on how to approach and manage SMIs effectively, summarized below.

Major Depressive Disorder

Medication. Moderate to severe depression often requires antidepressants, though they take a few weeks to show effects. There are various types of antidepressants, like SSRIs (such as Prozac or Zoloft) or SNRIs (such as Effexor or Cymbalta), which are standard first-line treatments for depression. Other types of medications, such as lithium, antipsychotics, thyroid hormones, and stimulants, are sometimes combined with antidepressants to enhance their effects. If the first medication doesn't work, there's a good chance that another might be more effective. In treatment-resistant cases, options such as electroconvulsive therapy (ECT), transcranial magnetic stimulation (TMS), and ketamine or esketamine may be considered. These alternatives have progressed significantly and are safe.

Psychotherapy. Various forms of psychotherapy can be effective in treating major depressive disorder. Two well-known approaches are CBT and interpersonal therapy (IPT). CBT focuses on challenging negative thoughts and beliefs, while IPT focuses on relationship issues. Research has shown that both options can match the effectiveness of medication, especially for mild to moderate depression. A combination of medication and therapy can enhance treatment outcomes.

Note that major depressive disorder may require hospitalization if your loved one's symptoms become life-threatening or debilitating.

Bipolar Disorder

Medication. There are numerous medication options to treat bipolar disorder. Treatments typically include lithium and certain anticonvulsants to help stabilize mood. Antipsychotics may be used during mania because they tend to act quickly and have high efficacy. Some antipsychotics also treat depression. Traditional antidepressants may be part of the treatment plan for bipolar disorder, but their use is debated, as they may trigger a manic episode and they may be less effective for bipolar disorder than for major depressive disorder.

Early diagnosis and treatment lead to better outcomes, helping prevent more complex symptoms and treatment resistance. Relapses are common, so ongoing vigilance is needed.

Psychotherapy. Various types of psychotherapy can be effective in treating bipolar disorder, including CBT, family-focused therapy (FFT), and interpersonal and social rhythm therapy (IPSRT). CBT, again, seeks to change maladaptive thinking and behavioral patterns. FFT involves psychoeducation, communication enhancement training, and training in problem-solving skills. Finally, IPSRT helps improve medication adherence, manage stressful life events, and reduce disruptions in "social rhythms" or patterns of daily habit.

Schizophrenia

Schizophrenia has both positive and negative symptoms, as discussed in chapter 1, Understanding Your Situation. We often associate schizophrenia only with positive symptoms, which we in turn make the focus of medical treatment. However, the treatment of negative symptoms and cognitive impairments—like memory, attention, planning, and solving problems—is critically important to long-term functioning as well. Unfortunately, cognition and negative symptoms can be more difficult to treat, and they sometimes persist even with treatment.

Comprehensive and integrated treatment—treatment including both medication and psychotherapy—is the most effective approach to treating schizophrenia. With treatment, most symptoms can greatly improve, and the likelihood of recurring episodes is reduced.

Medication. Antipsychotic drugs are the most common medical treatment for schizophrenia. They regulate brain chemicals affecting thought, emotion, and behavior. Mood stabilizers and antidepressants may also be used to address co-occurring conditions such as depression, sleep disturbances, and anxiety disorder. Long-acting injectable (LAI) medications are sometimes recommended to overcome adherence challenges.

Potential side effects such as tardive dyskinesia (TD) and weight gain should be monitored and addressed to improve treatment adherence and outcomes. TD involves involuntary facial and body movements that might become permanent. Weight gain is also a significant concern. The increased risks of cardiovascular problems and strokes are often overlooked when treating schizophrenia.

Psychotherapy. The psychotherapeutic treatment of schizophrenia often involves a range of complementary approaches including therapy, education, and support programs.

Therapy can help people develop coping skills. For example, CBT can address both positive and negative symptoms and help explore and reexamine thoughts and perceptions. It can also help support cognitive abilities. Other forms of therapy, like dialectical behavior therapy (DBT), discussed further below, can also help.

Other complementary strategies can also improve quality of life, promote personal strength, and treatment adherence. Cognitive remediation programs include computer-based training exercises and one-on-one sessions with a trained expert. Social skills training can enhance personal interactions. Supported work programs (discussed in chapter 7) can also have meaningful impact on quality of life.

There are also many non-medication treatments, such as ECT and newer forms of brain stimulation that can often help address symptoms of schizophrenia.

Other Treatment Considerations

The following are additional considerations that may be relevant to developing a treatment plan best suited to your loved one's needs.

Substance Use Disorders

People with SMIs often experience co-occurring SUDs. Integrated treatment involves addressing both the SMI and the SUD in a comprehensive manner, including their interactions. This approach is considered the gold standard and is essential for effective treatment.

If your loved one struggles with both SUD and SMI, seek a psychiatrist trained in addiction medicine who can offer integrated treatment. This specialized approach can better meet your loved one's needs.

Your loved one may be reluctant to stop using substances, and not see substance use as a problem. Optimal treatment aims for recovery and abstinence, but some experts suggest a "harm reduction approach," allowing monitored use of substances rather than complete abstinence. Studies show that this approach may work better for mild to moderate, but not severe, SUD. It is also possible for someone to start with a harm reduction approach and then transition to abstinence depending on their individual circumstances.

Cultural Competency

A culturally competent mental health professional understands how culture, race, ethnicity, sexual orientation, and gender identity can impact a person's well-being. They use this insight to tailor treatments to individual needs and backgrounds, thereby enhancing the effectiveness of therapy.

These professionals can build trust, demonstrate empathy, and facilitate open communication, even when language barriers exist. This approach is essential because individuals from diverse backgrounds often face higher rates of mental health issues and reduced access to treatment.

As mentioned earlier, when meeting with a potential provider, ask how they plan to incorporate your loved one's cultural background and beliefs into the treatment plan.

Trauma-Informed Care

Many people have experienced trauma in their lives, which can increase the risk of developing mental health issues and intensify existing conditions. Examples of trauma include physical, emotional, or sexual abuse and physical or emotional neglect. Trauma can also lead to anxiety, mood disturbances, and SUDs.

Trauma-informed care establishes safety, prevents re-traumatization, and promotes education. It can improve treatment outcomes and support your loved one's recovery.

Other Healthcare Providers

Other healthcare providers, beyond psychiatrists and PCPs, can play a crucial role in your loved one's treatment journey. These include psychiatric nurse practitioners, psychotherapists, and certified peer specialists.

PSYCHIATRIC NURSE PRACTITIONERS

These registered nurses and advanced practice registered nurses can often provide some basic primary care services as well as render psychiatric treatment. They work in a wide range of settings, often have specialized training, and are subject to licensing and credentialing standards. They can prescribe medication, often provide psychotherapy, and are more accessible and cost-effective than seeing a psychiatrist.

PSYCHOTHERAPISTS

A psychotherapist (or therapist) is any clinician who practices therapy, including social workers, psychologists, nurses, and certain psychiatrists. They can offer diagnoses and various forms of psychotherapy, though they don't prescribe medication unless they hold a medical license or appropriate nursing qualifications.

If your loved one is considering seeing a psychotherapist, inquire about their credentials and expertise to ensure they meet your loved one's needs.

PROFESSIONAL PEER SUPPORT

Certified Peer Specialists (CPSs) are people in recovery who help other peers reach recovery. They can help peers manage mental illness, trauma, substance use, and comorbid physical illnesses. They may also help with other recovery-oriented goals, such as education, employment, housing, and social connectedness. CPSs primarily work in the public sector.

Research by Dr. Chyrell Bellamy and her colleagues at Yale University shows that peer services have a positive impact on levels of hope, empowerment, and quality of life (Bellamy, Schmutte, and Davidson 2017).

Family Involvement

We now shift from discussing the potential role of individual healthcare providers to family-oriented interventions that can enhance education, support, and recovery.

Family Therapy

Family therapy is a form of psychological counseling focused on the family unit and designed to enhance communication among family members and resolve conflicts. It can be especially helpful to address problems with communication. It is typically facilitated by a psychologist, clinical social worker, or other therapy professional. These professionals hold advanced degrees. In the US, they may be accredited by the American Association for Marriage and Family Therapy.

Family therapy is typically a short-term approach. It may involve the entire family or select members. Skills learned during sessions can strengthen family bonds and help navigate difficult times, even once therapy concludes.

Privacy Rights

Gaining access to your loved one's treatment information can be beneficial for effective caregiving. However, this access requires consent due to privacy laws like the Health Insurance Portability and Accountability Act (HIPAA). Respect your loved one's autonomy and privacy when requesting access. If your loved one is a child, you will still want to exercise caution and care for their privacy to preserve trust when accessing information.

Healthcare providers can reveal a loved one's healthcare information when they receive verbal or written consent from them. In certain situations, the provider may also be comfortable sharing information when:

- You are present in your loved one's consultation

- A provider has concerns about your loved one's safety or potential harm to others

- They determine that your loved one lacks decision-making capacity

It is important to address these considerations promptly. A healthcare power of attorney (POA) or psychiatric advance directive (PAD—see the next section for more) typically grants a caregiver access to the patient's medical and mental health records.

Note that for college students, the Family Education Rights and Privacy (FERPA) might apply. FERPA empowers students to control who accesses their records and guarantees confidentiality. FERPA is especially notable since 75 percent of mental illnesses emerge by age twenty-four (NAMI n.d.). If your loved one is in this category, it's crucial to encourage them to sign a waiver before symptoms arise to ensure you are informed, should concerns arise while they're away from home.

Psychiatric Advance Directive

It's prudent to plan for and discuss a potential crisis with your loved one in advance. Completing a PAD offers an excellent opportunity for such conversations. A PAD is a legal document that enables your loved one to express their treatment preferences before a crisis occurs:

treatments to be administered or avoided, medications to use or not use, preferred hospitals and doctors, emergency contacts, and even the potential appointment of a decision-maker on their behalf.

You and your loved one can use standard forms to create your own PAD, ensuring you're well-prepared (see the National Resource Center on Psychiatric Advance Directives website for more information). Lawyers can also help you create your PAD. It's crucial to share the PAD with family members and healthcare providers.

Conservatorship

Sometimes when a condition deteriorates or leads to a crisis, it may call into question the loved one's capacity to make informed decisions in major life areas such as health and finances. If that occurs, you, a doctor, or another trusted friend or family member might pursue guardianship or conservatorship. In this process, a judge determines whether to grant decision-making authority.

Alternatives to Hospitalization

In a crisis, there are potential alternative forms of intervention that might avoid reaching an emergency level requiring hospitalization.

PEER RESPITE

Peer respite is a voluntary and short-term program, usually available in larger cities, designed to offer crisis support within a community-based environment. It is intended to feel like a home rather than a clinical setting. These facilities are run by peers who share similar experiences. Peer respite might help you and your loved one manage an emerging crisis before it escalates into an emergency. You may want to discuss this option with your loved one's healthcare provider in terms of its appropriateness for their given level of symptoms. According to one study, the odds of using inpatient services or emergency services after using these services are about 70 percent lower among respite users (Croft and Isvan 2015).

OUTPATIENT PROGRAM

Many hospitals offer intensive adult outpatient (IOPs) or partial hospital programs (PHP). In these programs, people live at home while actively participating in various services typically for about two to six weeks. They also often provide a transition after an inpatient stay. Hospital staff supervise the program and seek to determine if a patient's condition is severe enough to necessitate more intensive care, such as in cases of acute suicidality. These programs are also designed to aid a person's reintegration into the community and to prevent or minimize future hospital admissions.

Emergencies

If a mental illness cannot be effectively addressed through outpatient care, it might be deemed an emergency. A key determiner would be whether there's a risk or actual attempt of suicide, self-harm, or harm to others.

An emergency response, as is common in these situations, can be a frightening and traumatic experience for your loved one and you. Have a plan in place in case of emergency situations.

988

The 988 Suicide and Crisis Lifeline in the US offers three-digit telephone and text access to trained responders who offer compassionate response to callers in crisis. These responders listen, provide support, and direct individuals to relevant resources. Note a small percentage of Lifeline calls require activation of the 911 system when there is imminent risk to someone's life that cannot be reduced during the Lifeline call.

Crisis Intervention Teams

An alternative to calling 988 during a mental health crisis may be contacting a Crisis Intervention Team (CIT). According to CIT International (n.d.), a CIT is a "community partnership of law enforcement, mental health and addiction professionals, individuals who live with mental illness and/or addiction disorders, their caregivers, and advocates." This network operates in more than 2,700 communities across the US.

Alternatively, a Mobile Crisis Team (MCT) consisting of mental health professionals can provide assistance and medical evaluations.

Explore any CITs or MCTs in your local area and have their contact details ready in case of a potential crisis. Preparing this information beforehand can be quite helpful.

911

Dialing 911 in the US is the most serious and potentially complex action to take. I (Katherine) was upset with my partner for years because they called 911 during a difficult time. I held them responsible for my hospital stay. I felt ashamed that my neighbors might have witnessed me in crisis. Fearing a recurrence of this, I hesitated seeking help, which unfortunately contributed to two more hospitalizations.

As I recovered, I began to understand my partner's position at that time. Looking back, I believe we could have managed the crisis differently and possibly avoided calling 911 if we'd been prepared or had accessed other options had we known about them.

Hospitalization

A patient might be admitted to the hospital either voluntarily or involuntarily. The criteria for admission generally require that they pose a danger either to themself or others or are gravely impaired.

If a healthcare professional has recommended inpatient care, and you are unsure if that is the best next step, and circumstances are not urgent, consider seeking a second opinion from a psychiatrist about the viability of alternative treatment options. If hospitalization is determined to be the best step, your loved one will likely be taken to a psychiatric emergency room. It's worth noting that these rooms can be chaotic, and a shortage of available beds is common.

Once admitted, your loved one will receive continuous supervision and may undergo a seventy-two-hour hold to evaluate their condition. If further treatment is needed, they may be transferred to the inpatient unit.

Moving Forward

When planning treatment, consider your loved one's past psychiatric experiences and the potential course of their illness. Understanding these factors can help set realistic expectations and guide future interventions. It can help determine which treatment options and resources may be more effective in both crisis and non-crisis environments.

In the next chapter, we will discuss triggers: events and situations that can cause or exacerbate your loved one's mental illness symptoms. Being able to recognize and address triggers will be an important part of the treatment plan and goals you and your loved one will develop.

Identifying and Responding to Triggers

CHAPTER 6

A trigger, or stressor, is an event or situation that can lead to an emotional response, often adverse (though occasionally positive). In the context of mental health, triggers usually cause or worsen symptoms. Your understanding, awareness, and response to your loved one's triggers can play a critical role in helping them manage symptoms. This chapter will teach you about different types of triggers and strategies to respond constructively to, and even learn from, them.

Triggers, as the word suggests, are often the immediate cause, even source, of symptoms. If your loved one has an existing genetic susceptibility to mental health disorders, high stress can serve as a trigger, activating a psychiatric condition—especially if they lack effective stress management skills. Research has established this link for major depressive disorder (Kendler, Karlowski, and Prescott 1999), bipolar disorder (Koenders et al. 2014), and schizophrenia (Lecomte et al. 2019).

Triggers can also contribute to the onset or exacerbation of symptoms if your loved one already deals with a mental illness. In bipolar disorder, triggers can set in motion a hypomanic or manic episode. For schizophrenia, they might contribute to hallucinations and delusions. And for major depressive disorder, they can deepen the sense of depression.

Surprisingly, preparing for triggers is often overlooked in discussions of mental illness. There's a tendency to focus on what to do after a loved one has been triggered, at which point addressing symptoms may be harder. Identifying and seeking to prevent triggers can empower you and your loved one to reduce or even eliminate certain symptoms.

There are four main categories of mental health triggers: stigma, internal, external, and trauma. Any one of them can prompt the emergence of early warning signs signaling that your loved one is at risk of developing symptoms. For instance, a trigger could lead to physical reactions such as heavy breathing or sweating, or spark emotional reactions like feeling attacked, blamed, controlled, disrespected, hurt, or judged.

Stigma Triggers

The stigma of mental illness can be the most detrimental trigger. External events, or public stigma (judgment your loved one receives from others or the world around them), can irritate or anger them, potentially leading to an episode. Caregivers should be conscious of their own potential stigmatizing beliefs (e.g., depression is a personal weakness rather than an illness) that they might unwittingly impose on their loved one. Internal events, or self-stigma (judgments your loved one applies to themself), can also activate a range of emotions, which might trigger rumination, worsening and potentially activating symptoms.

One of the gravest consequences of stigma is that your loved one may choose not to seek services that might benefit them (Corrigan 2004), may become lax about medication adherence, or may otherwise not be able to fully engage in their care. Remember that the average time between the onset of symptoms and receiving treatment is approximately eleven years (NAMI n.d.). Many delay treatment or never access it. Such delayed intervention can exacerbate conditions, making them harder to manage and worsening health outcomes.

Stigma may also prevent your loved one from cultivating relationships, leading to withdrawal and isolation. Additionally, it might contribute to a reluctance to engage in other life activities essential to recovery, such as employment. Inaction may be the most detrimental impact of stigma. Remember that stigma is often based on ignorance or misinformation about mental illness and has little or no correspondence to reality.

Let's dive a little deeper into the two types of stigma.

Public Stigma

Public stigma is the type of stigma that most commonly comes to mind (Corrigan and Rao 2012). It refers to negative beliefs and biases that society largely projects onto groups with "devalued" characteristics, such as mental illness. These may include unfounded notions of people with SMIs as perilous, irresponsible, inept, untrustworthy, unpredictable, or inclined toward interpersonal conflict. Media portrayals that link baseless assumptions about mental health issues and public acts of violence exacerbate these biases.

As a caregiver, you play a crucial role in deflecting these distortions and supporting your loved one when they encounter such biases. When your loved one reveals they've been affected by public stigma, talk to them; help them work through it.

Self-Stigma

Most people with mental illness encounter public stigma at some point. It can come from friends, family, employers, or healthcare providers. But self-stigma—when people with mental illness develop negative self-perceptions or internalize society's negative stereotypes—can be particularly harmful.

Your loved one's sense of self-stigma will vary with their individual circumstances. But it often hinges on preexisting feelings of guilt and shame.

The Internalized Stigma Mental Illness Inventory-29 (ISMI-29; Ritsher, Otilingam, and Grajales 2003) measures self-stigma across five categories summarized below:

1. *Alienation:* This may lead your loved one to blame themself for their condition, feel embarrassed or inferior, and believe others misunderstand them. They may also feel their illness has disrupted or even destroyed their life.

2. *Stereotype endorsement:* Your loved one might internalize misconceptions associated with mental illness—like people with SMI are violent, cognitively impaired, unable to make reasoned decisions, or incapable of living a normal life. This may weaken their sense of self and confidence.

3. *Discrimination experience:* Feeling discriminated against, overlooked, or dismissed may lead your loved one to believe others are unwilling to form relationships with them. As a result,

they may feel unable to reach personal or professional goals—a big barrier to lasting recovery.

4. *Social withdrawal:* Your loved one may avoid close relationships and limit or avoid social interactions. Perhaps they feel like a burden or want to prevent embarrassment for themself or others.

5. *Stigma resistance:* Your loved one may protect themself from stigma by recognizing the value of people with SMI, embracing associations with others in similar situations, viewing mental illness as a source of resilience, and recognizing their potential for a fulfilling life.

Stigma can be amplified in many ways. Your loved one may generalize from their experiences of stigma. They may presume that even those who don't actively stigmatize are still biased (also called perceived stigma). They may also anticipate stigma.

As a caregiver, it's crucial for you to assume that your loved one is affected by and deeply influenced by stigma, even if they may not be consciously aware of it. Also, the emotional toll of self-stigma can be severe. It can wreck self-esteem, self-efficacy, and overall perspective on life and cause your loved one to avoid discussing their condition or seeking treatment. Therefore, recognizing and addressing self-stigma are critical to recovery.

When discussing self-stigma, respect how it affects your loved one emotionally, rather than dismissing their belief in these stereotypes. You should tell your loved one that stigma reflects false narratives and persuade your loved one to reject stigmatizing ideas because they have no basis in their individual truth.

EXERCISE: **Assessing Self-Stigma**

In chapter 7, Wellness Plan, you'll learn about emotion-focused coping, which will help you address your loved one's emotional reactions to triggers and underlying feelings and emotions linked to stigma. For now, now that you have learned about the different dimensions of self-stigma, ask your loved one the following questions to better understand how they are impacted by self-stigma:

- Do you ever blame yourself for your mental illness?

- Do you believe any of the common stereotypes of mental illness are accurate?

- Have you experienced discrimination or felt overlooked because of your mental illness?

- Are you withdrawing from social interactions or avoiding close relationships because of your mental illness?

- What strategies can we use to resist the negative effects of stigma?

Internal Triggers

Internal triggers are emotional responses, thoughts, and feelings sparked by present or past experiences that can lead to further, often negative, behaviors and emotional responses. Internal triggers can have a more significant impact than external triggers and are typically more common. They're often unpredictable and nonrecurring. And to some extent, they're unavoidable—it's simply not possible to prevent all thoughts, feelings, and emotional responses that lead to other challenging emotions and behaviors. An internal trigger can also precede an external one, making it more challenging to problem solve the external trigger. Therefore, you may need to address the internal trigger before turning your attention to the external trigger.

Here are common internal triggers and examples of why your loved one may be experiencing them and easy and quick ways to address them:

Depressed: Struggling with illness limitations → set and achieve reasonable goals

Embarrassed: "Inappropriate" behavior due to illness → reassure them that it was their illness; there's no need to apologize

Fearful: Of never getting better → show examples of recovery

Lonely: Battling social isolation → offer companionship and unwavering support

Stressed: By daily life with mental illness → help them learn self-care

Traumatized: By hospitalizations → explain it was necessary at the time

Worried: About recovery → reassure them: most people do recover

Note that many of these emotions may occur simultaneously, which can make it difficult to determine how to address them. The first step is to validate your loved one's emotions. Next, ask them how they're feeling, using active listening skills discussed more in the Talking About Mental Illness chapter (8). Then, ask them how you can help.

Anger

All the above emotions can express themselves in anger—they may be felt internally and suppressed until they eventually surface as anger. You may misinterpret this anger as directed toward you without apparent cause and react defensively; this misunderstanding can escalate into verbal conflicts or, at worst, physical ones.

It's especially valuable to cultivate your ability to observe and understand what your loved one is going through—and what you're going through—in any given moment, and to familiarize yourself with de-escalation techniques (as detailed in chapter 3).

You may feel like you're constantly tiptoeing around your loved one to avoid interactions that could be triggering. Familiarity with fundamental strategies to avoid and defuse emotionally charged situations can help you engage constructively with them while maintaining the calm.

Mourning a Former Self

Accepting mental illness can be challenging, leading to emotional distress akin to mourning. This struggle may persist for years, leading to deferred treatment and worsening outcomes. Acceptance comes with its own challenges. Most with mental illness wish to revert to their pre-diagnosis selves but must embrace their new life to achieve the best outcome.

Recognizing their condition may bring your loved one significant emotional distress that feels like mourning. Similarly, you might mourn the person and relationship you expected to have.

You must recognize that the illness poses challenges and requires adjustments, but your loved one's life with mental illness can be fulfilling and happy. So can yours.

EXERCISE: **Processing Loss**

Write or record answers to the following questions to begin processing how you feel:

- When did you and your loved one last feel mourning or grief related to your loved one's recovery?

- What losses were you mourning?

- What is different about how you think about the loss as time has passed?

Hopelessness

Hopelessness—the sense that the situation one is facing will not improve, and that there is nothing good coming in the future—can be one of the most devastating internal emotions. It can trigger a range of feelings, from sadness to anger to defeat and despair, which are significant hurdles to recovery. Hopelessness can also hinder your loved one's inclination to socialize, motivation to adhere to treatment, and more profoundly, their will to live. In severe cases, intense feelings of hopelessness have been shown to be significant predictors of suicidality (Beck, Brown, and Steer 1989). To pursue recovery, it's crucial to combat triggers that dampen morale and to nurture hope in your loved one. Maintaining hope, for both of you, fuels a commitment to the recovery journey.

Before reading on, take a moment to think or journal about the following question: What do or can you do to maintain hope in your loved one? And yourself?

External Triggers

External triggers arise from environmental factors or events. Life-altering events—like changes to living arrangements or family structures, or loss of a loved one—are among the most severe external triggers. They're difficult to navigate because they disrupt predictable routines and people often lack experience to address them. The most effective approach to managing these triggers may be to address the emotional response they evoke.

However, many external, often recurring, triggers can be anticipated and controlled with established coping strategies. Below are a few examples of common, everyday triggers that problem-focused coping strategies (discussed in the next chapter) can help mitigate. These strategies include actions that you as a caregiver can help with or practice.

Trigger	Problem-Focused Coping
Sleep too little	Practice sleep hygiene
Overweight	Find ways to make exercise more fun
Alcohol consumption	No socializing at bars
Told what to do	Caregiver avoids nagging
Accused of not trying hard enough	Caregiver expresses pride in loved one's effort
Stigmatized	Caregiver counters stigma with facts

Some external triggers, such as tragedies, are best addressed with emotion-focused coping strategies. The Holmes-Rahe Stress Inventory (Holmes and Rahe 1967) is a common instrument for measuring stress. It identifies forty-three external triggers for people in the general population.

These are also common triggers for people with SMI. External triggers include family, work, unemployment, school, changes to routine, other everyday events, and factors in your loved one's immediate physical or social environments. We'll discuss each one below.

Family

Family-related developments can be potent external triggers, often provoking significant emotional responses and behaviors. Leading family-related external triggers include the death of a spouse or other close family member or friend, divorce or separation, marriage, family illness, domestic conflict, a child leaving home, in-law troubles, and changes in family socialization.

Work

Events in professional life can cause significant emotional responses. These triggers include terminations, retirements, transition to different career paths, and noteworthy changes in responsibilities, such as promotions or demotions. Outstanding personal achievements can also play a role, as well as challenges involving supervisors, colleagues, or subordinates, or substantial changes in working hours or conditions.

Financial Issues

Financial control can be a significant concern in the caregiver-loved one relationship. Issues with employment can make your loved one financially dependent on you, which can trigger relationship issues. It's especially challenging for caregivers with limited incomes. Studies show that nearly half of people with SMI are unemployed (Luciano and Meara 2014), with many relying on caregivers for financial support. This dependency can strain household dynamics and lead to caregiver resentment, particularly as people with SMI aspire for independence.

Your loved one may also struggle with managing their finances—perhaps making imprudent purchases that lead you to control their access to money. It's advisable to anticipate these issues and establish mutual agreements to regulate spending. It can be helpful to have such discussions before they are necessary. For example, a caregiver and loved one may agree that the loved one gives their credit card to the caregiver if their spending exceeds an agreed amount. Consequences for not adhering to the mutual agreement should be spelled out in advance. Using the same example, if the loved one exceeds the agreed spending limit and refuses to give the card to their caregiver, the caregiver may contact a psychiatrist for an appointment. Attempting to restrict access to funds or dictate spending can often lead to confrontations and power struggles, making it important to find collaborative solutions.

School

School-related stressors include beginning or ceasing schooling, changing schools, and poor grades. Refusal to go to school sometimes occurs in youth with an emerging SMI. It may escalate into tension and struggle within the home that may be difficult to remedy if you don't recognize it's happening and help your loved one through it.

Changes to Routine

External factors that disturb regular sleep patterns can exacerbate certain types of SMI. In bipolar disorder, for example, occasional evening shifts or nonstandard work hours may trigger mood-related symptoms. Travel across time zones can disrupt mood stability, as can changes to daily routines. Alcohol and substance use, interruptions in medication, and medication side effects contribute to mood disruptions.

Environmental Conditions

Understanding the environment in which your loved one lives, works, socializes, and otherwise interacts with other people is crucial in addressing their overall well-being, both physically and emotionally. By paying attention to these social factors, you are better positioned to enhance your loved one's mental health and even prevent symptoms. Poverty stands out as one of the most significant determinants of mental well-being. Economic hardships can lead to various symptoms and make it difficult to access quality care for mental health issues. Therefore, helping your loved one seek employment opportunities, access relevant financial support programs, and plan their personal finances may contribute significantly to their well-being.

Other Everyday Events

Everyday-event triggers should be addressed as quickly as possible as part of a wellness plan. Chapter 7 will discuss how to manage some of the more common everyday triggers, such as relationship conflicts, work stress, school stress, sleep interruptions, substance use, poor diet, and lack of exercise.

Trauma Triggers

A trauma trigger is often an external trigger that evokes a person's memories or feelings of past traumatic events. A traumatic event is a drastic, shocking, or life-threatening experience that leaves lasting physical or emotional effects. Triggers that stem from trauma may develop in childhood and be long lasting.

There are specific treatment approaches to address trauma triggers. You should offer to help your loved one explore these approaches with their doctor or therapist. Ultimately, you can play a valuable role helping recognize and address trauma triggers in your loved one with a clinician's guidance.

Hospitalizations

Mental illnesses sometimes lead to hospitalization. For many with SMI, it may be their first significant encounter with treatment. Unfortunately, hospitalization tends to exacerbate patients' emotions, intensifying feelings of depression and anxiety (Alzahrani 2021). Hospitalization, especially when it occurs involuntarily, can be exceedingly traumatic. The process of involuntary hospitalization often starts with a visible police response along with EMTs and may involve physical or chemical restraints. The experience can feel akin to imprisonment, instilling deep fear in your loved one of future hospitalization. This can potentially strain the caregiver relationship and lead to deferred treatments and otherwise preventable future crises. So, when discussing potential hospitalization with your loved one, it's critically important for you to convey an unwavering commitment to their safety and fundamental well-being.

In the event of a mental health crisis where your loved one poses a risk to themself or others, you should make every effort to persuade them to undergo a proper clinical evaluation. If hospitalization is recommended, for your loved one to do so voluntarily may be less traumatic. Voluntary hospitalization follows a more discrete and typically less stressful admission process. Additionally, it's ideal to have in place a PAD, as discussed in chapter 5, to guide such situations. You should offer to help your loved one navigate the different options to mitigate the potential stress and trauma of hospitalization. You and your loved one want to control that process to the extent that you can.

Negative Prognosis

Receiving a negative prognosis can be profoundly distressing and cause your loved one to resist the diagnosis and treatment. Mental health providers may knowingly or not perpetuate stigma if they deliver bad news without fostering some sense of hope. You may need to help your loved one get past a poorly delivered prognosis by remaining positive and hopeful and reinforcing your support.

Addressing Triggers

While you can prevent some triggering events, you won't be able to eliminate triggers from your loved one's life. The most effective thing you can do is to learn about triggers and anticipate them. Understanding the nature of triggers—their causes, and how they impact your loved one—is key to helping your loved one manage them.

The following are key characteristics of triggers to keep in mind:

- Triggers are closely tied to change—which can include positive events, like marriage, rather than exclusively negative occurrences, such as job loss. This principle also applies to emotional responses; triggers can evoke both positive and negative emotions.

- If your loved one is exposed to triggers while experiencing symptoms, they may exhibit greater vulnerability and more intense emotional reactions.

- Triggers have the potential to impair judgment. Your loved one may lack insight into their own reactions.

- Your loved one's specific triggers are highly individual and likely to differ from those of other people with mental illness, while having many common features.

- Typically, triggers emerge gradually, although they can also manifest suddenly. Furthermore, one trigger may set off another. Or they may occur in tandem.

- Triggers are an integral part of life. Mental health recovery is not necessarily about avoiding them but about effectively managing their impact.

- Some triggers are foreseeable.

- Your loved one's capacity to manage triggers can fluctuate from day to day.

- Your loved one may exhibit more pronounced physical and emotional reactions to triggers that also affect people without SMI.

- Your loved one's reaction to a trigger can range from relatively minor to severe, including intense outburst of emotion. They may have an episode or experience feelings of being over-whelmed, powerless, fearful, unloved, or vulnerable, among other negative emotions.

The following are key behaviors that you should avoid in responding to your loved one's triggers:

- Presuming that you fully comprehend your loved one's physical or emotional responses to triggers.

- Implying that your loved one, when triggered, is exaggerating a physical condition, exhibiting excessive emotional reactions, being "too sensitive," or behaving irrationally. This is invalidating behavior.

- Discouraging your loved one from taking the risks necessary for recovery in a bid to keep their stress levels low to avoid triggering them. You can discuss your concerns with your loved one openly, but it's important to allow them to decide on the appropriate course of action. Risks are often essential for personal growth.

"Positive" Triggers

Thus far, our emphasis has primarily been on triggers that have adverse consequences. But certain triggers can lead to positive outcomes. For instance, anger can drive you to transform challenging interpersonal relationships or external circumstances. Or, if you lose your job, this setback might motivate you to actively seek out more fulfilling employment opportunities. Stress can also be a force for good; for example, the stress of a test you want to do well on may motivate you to study. This form of stress is commonly referred to as "eustress." It can also serve as one of the forces that encourages PTG (post-traumatic growth).

Recognizing that triggers can lead to positive outcomes can help your loved one cope with them. You can help them find the positive possibilities in certain triggers. This reframing can help your loved one address the trigger more constructively.

Post-traumatic Growth

Some people, in response to a traumatic event, find they can maintain hope and uncover meaning in life despite the pain, loss, and suffering. According to Tedeschi and Calhoun (2004), these responses can reflect PTG: positive transformation that can emerge from grappling with profoundly challenging life crises. Examples they identify of this transformation include "increased appreciation for life in general, more meaningful interpersonal relationships, increased sense of personal strength, changed priorities, and a richer existential and spiritual life."

You can help your loved one recognize the possibility for personal growth over time from a traumatic experience. You can encourage your loved one to examine their life as they advance in the recovery process, which can foster resilience and enable them to transcend their mental illness.

Preparing a Plan for Triggers

You can take proactive steps following an episode to better anticipate potential triggers in the future. These steps include:

- Reflecting on the past—the same triggers that precipitated a previous episode are the most likely to do so again

- Analyzing recurring patterns—your loved one may consistently be triggered by the same factors; try to discern the patterns

- Establishing guidelines based on patterns—prior experiences can help you determine how long to wait before seeking assistance

As the expert on your loved one's triggers, you can proactively address them and develop a comprehensive plan including coping skills and involvement of healthcare providers. Ultimately, you and your loved one should develop a comprehensive plan to address known triggers, including specific plans to involve healthcare providers such as a psychiatrist for medication adjustments or therapy with a therapist. Such a plan should also include a set of coping skills and tools that can be employed at the very onset of feeling triggered.

EXERCISE: Addressing Triggers

With your loved one, complete the following steps:

1.   Identify external and internal triggers based on past experiences both actual and probable.

2.   Consider: Which events led to the external and internal triggers?

3.   Identify the best way to address triggers based on this chapter and the Wellness Plan chapter.

4.   In identifying the trigger, assign responsibilities for how the caregiver, loved one, or healthcare provider can each best address and help in managing specific triggers.

5.   Also develop rules of thumb on what action needs to be taken, based on severity and duration of each trigger. Assign responsibilities for caregiver, loved one, and healthcare provider.

6.   Identify early warning signs connected to each trigger.

7.   Identify early warning signs connected to each symptom.

Moving Forward

In the next chapter, we'll discuss additional ways to address the most common external triggers. We'll also offer problem-focused coping strategies to prevent them from reoccurring, and emotion-focused coping strategies to help your loved one get through them when they're present.

CHAPTER 7 — **Wellness Plan**

This chapter provides you strategies to help your loved one manage triggers and maintain wellness. Both managing triggers and promoting wellness can mitigate stressors that could otherwise exacerbate psychiatric symptoms. We'll explore what's effective in stress management and what's not. Both are valuable to understand because effective coping strategies involve encouraging positive behaviors and avoiding certain activities. You will gain practical insights into a range of stress management strategies, including medication, therapy, communication, and a holistic wellness plan. This chapter also highlights the interconnected nature of all dimensions of wellness in promoting positive mental health outcomes.

Comprehensive Approaches

There are many strategies to address triggers and promote well-being. Two broad categories are "emotion-focused coping" (EFC) and "problem-focused coping" (PFC) (Lazarus and Folkman 1984). EFC addresses emotional reactions to triggers, while PFC seeks concrete solutions to resolve problems.

Emotion-focused coping is crucial in dealing with major external events and internal triggers. These situations are often unpredictable, arising from non-recurring, one-off events, and may be unavoidable. Cognitive limitations (e.g., hallucinations) and intense emotional responses can also make it challenging to effectively employ problem-focused coping in these circumstances. Rumination on emotional thoughts, common in SMI, further complicates matters, contributing to the development or worsening of depression and other conditions.

Problem-focused coping is typically employed in situations where external triggers can be resolved. These triggers are often predictable, recurring, and, to some extent, avoidable. They're typically not life-changing. The key aspect of PFC is finding means to resolve the problem, which subsequently address the emotional triggers associated with it. PFC becomes essential in navigating challenges that, with prior experience, can be tackled systematically, providing a more structured and problem-solving-oriented response to stressors.

Specific Approaches

There are several specific EFC and PFC strategies that may be grouped into four categories, namely medication, therapy, communication, and wellness plan.

Medication

Adhering to a medication regimen can aid significantly in managing triggers and promoting well-being. You can support adherence by helping your loved one understand the medication's importance, addressing obstacles like complex dosing regimens or side effects, providing daily reminders, or setting up a system for reminders like daily alarms or notifications. If your loved one permits it, you can also help communicate with the prescribing professional to address issues and gather more information. Be careful about sharing medication information from other sources that is not confirmed. Medication can also be incorporated into a behavioral contract (which we'll discuss later in this chapter).

Medication may also relieve stress. Since we're not psychiatrists, we asked Joseph Goldberg, a leading SMI psychiatrist, to share his insights on medication.

According to Goldberg, effective medications for SMI should ideally help loved ones manage their emotional reactions to stressful experiences. When triggers evoke intense feelings of anxiety, certain medicines may be helpful on an as-needed basis. Minor tranquilizers such as Xanax and Valium may not be ideal long-term choices as they can be habit-forming and abusable, but they may have some value when used sparingly. Some atypical antipsychotics can be helpful to reduce feelings of emotional distress, particularly at low doses. Some mood stabilizers such as valproate or lamotrigine, taken on a daily basis, have demonstrated value to reduce anxiety symptoms. Gabapentin is sometimes used either for as-needed or daily management of anxiety symptoms. Finally, certain antihistamines such as hydroxyzine also can be safe options for breakthrough anxiety on an as-needed basis. Sometimes, if "stress" points to an underlying anxiety disorder, daily treatment with medication such as a serotonergic antidepressant may help prevent flares.

Talk to your loved one about how they feel about medication and the possible benefits, and encourage them to speak to their psychiatrist and ask them for their recommendation on the best medication strategy. If your loved one is reluctant, they may be experiencing side effects, feel medications don't work, be discouraged by stigma, or even feel they don't need medication. Try to find out the source of their reluctance and address it. Encourage them to explore and discuss their ambivalence in therapy as well.

Therapy

Encouraging loved ones to see therapists, exploring different therapies, and applying techniques collaboratively can help more effectively manager triggers. You and your loved one might consider specific therapeutic approaches like CBT and DBT. CBT can help your loved one reframe their ideas and beliefs and develop alternative points of view. DBT strategies can help them regulate negative emotions and tolerate uncomfortable feelings.

Communication

Effective communication is essential to helping your loved one manage triggers. Chapter 8, Talking About Mental Illness, discusses many communication strategies. To help your loved one manage their triggers, try expressing empathy, ensuring your loved one feels heard, involving them in decision-making, understanding their needs, developing collaborative plans, addressing misunderstandings, and apologizing when necessary.

Use triggering events in your interactions with each other as learning experiences. You, like your loved one, are human and may be triggered as easily as *they* are. Sometimes their triggered behavior may even trigger you in turn. For example, if your loved one refuses suggestions or recommendations that seem reasonable, you may feel overwhelmed or exasperated.

Ultimately, as part of your wellness plan, figure out what's triggering to each of you, and identify ways to manage these triggers. This can involve you and your loved one sharing the other's actions and negative responses—when you're both calm. It may also help if you both apologize for triggering behaviors, even if the triggering was unintentional. It's important for you both to recognize that behavior that's triggering is typically unintentionally so.

It can be helpful to create a behavioral contract (see the exercise at the end of this chapter). This contract can incentivize you both to avoid situations that might be triggering you, such as medication nonadherence.

Also speak to others in your loved one's life who may be triggering them. You might let them know that their behavior can be upsetting (sharing only as much as your loved one permits). And when you're all together, you can act as a buffer for your loved one, diverting conversation from triggering topics. You might also gently discourage your loved one from spending time with people who may be bad for their mental health.

Wellness Plan

A wellness plan, like any other plan, begins with identifying the goals to work toward. It's important to understand your loved one's desires to best support them. Like caregivers often do, you may be most focused on getting your loved one to accept and adhere to treatment for their illness. But your loved one might focus on a broader set of life considerations, such as employment, relationships, and community involvement. Working with your loved one to identify their needs and desires can help you set well-informed goals for your plan. You may even discover that what you want and what they want are the same.

You should reinforce that treatment and adherence are essential to achieving these life goals, as they'll likely be. You'll also want to work with your loved one to develop a robust regimen that addresses triggers and supports overall wellness. Ultimately, your plan should allow your loved one to grow as a person and not just address or avoid episodes.

Building Your Own Wellness Plan—Eight Dimensions of Wellness

To help you and your loved one develop your own wellness plan tailored to your needs, we are sharing a potential framework—The Eight Dimensions of Wellness is a wellness model proposed by Swarbrick (2012) that's focused on building strength and resilience. It emphasizes that the dimensions are interconnected, and each has the potential to impact mental health positively or adversely. You'll find it useful in helping your loved one (and nurturing your own wellness, which mustn't be overlooked). We discuss each of these dimensions below.

Emotional Wellness

Emotional wellness can help you address a wide range of internal and external stressors and promote general well-being. The following strategies can benefit emotional wellness:

Mindfulness: Practicing mindfulness through meditation enhances self-awareness, reduces stress, and aids in emotion regulation. Mindfulness-based techniques can be particularly beneficial to people with psychotic disorders, though they can be challenging for those who struggle with rumination or sustained attention.

Journaling: Journaling can help manage immediate emotions and promote reflection, which can lead to better problem-solving. It helps control symptoms, recognize triggers, and identify negative thoughts and behaviors.

Positive self-affirmations: Self-affirmations boost self-esteem, counter negative distortions, and foster a positive self-image.

Radical acceptance: Radical acceptance, a DBT approach, encourages recognizing and accepting challenging circumstances that cannot be changed immediately (McKay, Wood, and Brantley 2019). Your loved one—and you—have the choice to either agonize over things they can't change or accept them as they are to move forward. Like many people, your loved one might require gentle encouragement to move on.

Fact-checking: Fact-checking is a basic and fundamental strategy for deciding if the way we feel aligns with objective reality. Facts are pieces of information that have no emotional content in themselves because they're simply true or false, with no judgment attached. And the ways we feel don't necessarily reflect the facts of a situation. Encouraging your loved one to fact-check can be a useful and compassionate way to help free them from painful emotions or ideas that may not be grounded in truth. Your loved one or you may, for instance, misinterpret the remarks someone has made about a situation.

Cognitive distortions: You can apply CBT's cognitive distortions framework to identify and challenge faulty thinking patterns (Beck 2020). Examples of cognitive distortions, drawn from Beck, include all-or-nothing thinking, catastrophizing, disqualifying the positive, emotional reasoning, labeling, personalization, and "should" and "must" statements. Addressing these distortions in your loved one's thinking, or yours, contributes to improved emotional wellness:

- All-or-nothing thinking (black and white thinking): perceiving situations in binary extremes instead of recognizing a range of possibilities

- Catastrophizing (fortune-telling): predicting the future negatively without considering more likely outcomes, often magnifying potential problems

- Disqualifying the positive: unreasonably convincing oneself that positive experiences, deeds, or qualities are not meaningful

- Emotional reasoning: believing something is true based on a feeling while neglecting or dismissing evidence to the contrary

- Labeling: attaching fixed labels to oneself or others without considering evidence that might reasonably lead to a less-extreme conclusion

- Personalization: blaming oneself for the negative behaviors of others, without considering more plausible explanations for that behavior

- "Should" and "must" statements: having a rigid and fixed idea of how you or others should behave

Reframing: Reshaping automatic negative thoughts into positive perceptions can greatly benefit emotional well-being, for you and your loved one. For example, you might shift from thinking "Nothing will ever be the same" to "Maybe something positive can come from this."

Emotional Support Animals: pet ownership can reduce feelings of isolation and loneliness (Wood et al. 2015). Pets are an important, trusted, and consistent source of unconditional love and affection. They intuitively provide this in times of need, and they can be a helpful distraction from ruminations on negative thoughts, including suicidal ideation. They are also accorded certain privileges under the law.

Financial Wellness

Financial stress is prevalent among households dealing with SMI. Many adult children with SMI—64 percent according to one study—are financially dependent on family and friends due to unemployment or underemployment (National Alliance for Caregiving 2016). You can help your loved one reduce financial stress by encouraging them to clarify financial goals, consider work, or come up with a financial plan. This may include creating a personal budget, with savings and investment objectives. Where financial assistance is needed, you can help your loved one explore relevant government benefits like Supplemental Security Income (SSI), Social Security Disability Insurance (SSDI), Medicaid and Medicare,

Veteran Affairs benefits, Supplemental Nutrition Assistance Program (SNAP, formerly known as food stamps), and public housing programs.

You can also help your loved one with monitoring spending and financial accounts if it's acceptable to them. You might formalize this by becoming their representative payee or conservator, but this isn't always necessary. Other financial tools that are available to help you assist your loved one include view-only account access or prepaid debit cards with customizable spending limits.

Your loved one may feel a sense of shame if they're unable to manage their finances or require financial assistance. You must help them recognize that their circumstances are a result of their illness, there's no shame in getting needed help, and they can improve their financial health. Otherwise, this shame may create a barrier to accessing the support and resources they need.

Occupational Wellness

Employment is considered by many to be the most important factor in mental health recovery. Secure income will often determine if your loved one is able to be financially independent. But people with SMI may face barriers like treatment-related issues, work history gaps, and low self-esteem. You can help address these barriers by providing material assistance and a supportive home environment as your loved one explores their options for employment. Be aware of any sense of shame your loved one may feel. They may compare their employment status to others like classmates and friends whom they may view to be "ahead" of them. It's worth reminding your loved one that whatever setbacks they've faced are due to the illness and they can succeed by focusing on their long-term wellness.

You can learn more about your loved one's career interests and help them search for job options, complete applications, prepare for interviews, and explore supported employment programs. These programs are often offered through government agencies such as community behavioral health centers, as well as Clubhouses. Their goal is to help people with mental illness find and keep meaningful jobs in the community.

One approach is Individual Placement and Support (IPS), which helps people with mental illness find competitive employment while receiving ongoing individualized long-term support. You can also encourage your loved one to seek volunteer opportunities as a way to build experience and obtain references, which can help in the search for paid work.

Understanding the Americans with Disabilities Act (ADA), which mandates accommodations for people with disabilities, can also be empowering. Some who receive disability benefits wish to work but fear ending up worse off financially by losing benefits as a result. But those who receive disability benefits can often work part-time and continue to receive government benefits. It may also be an option for your loved one to transition away from disability benefits if they feel confident enough in part-time work to move to full-time.

Finally, work is one of many variables for achieving and maintaining wellness. You should reinforce with your loved one that healthy work-life balance is always important for good mental health.

Physical Wellness

Physical and mental health are highly connected. SMIs cause symptoms and behaviors that negatively impact physical health, which can contribute to mental health issues. As a caregiver, you can help your loved one make improvements in physical health that can positively impact their mental illness journey.

SLEEP

Many people with SMI struggle with sleep as a symptom of or because of medication side effects, other medical conditions, or poor sleep hygiene. Sleep disturbances are linked to stress and can exacerbate mental health conditions. Insomnia or other difficulties sleeping may signal a mental health episode. Sleep disturbance is a key symptom of bipolar disorder and can trigger an episode. It's also a common sign of mania, when not followed by fatigue the next day. People with depression often have trouble falling or staying asleep, but also experience fatigue. People with schizophrenia also typically experience sleep abnormalities, often preceding illness onset or worsening of psychotic symptoms.

Your loved one's sleep patterns can be invaluable information to you as a caregiver. They can signal to you and your loved one to take action to avoid the onset or worsening of a mental health episode. If you notice a change in your loved one's sleep, you can share your observation with them and remind them of the potential significance. They might then adjust their routine to address the cause, if it's known, and otherwise improve sleep routines and hygiene. They may also consult their psychiatrist or other doctor for guidance or a prescription for a sleep medication.

EXERCISE

Exercise is helpful for enhancing mood as well as physical well-being.

Many studies show that exercise reduces symptoms of depression. In people with schizophrenia, exercise has been shown to improve both positive and negative symptoms as well as overall quality of life. Similarly in bipolar disorder, exercise can have a beneficial effect on mood and physical well-being.

Factors such as sedentary lifestyle and smoking status may discourage some people with SMI from engaging in exercise regimen schedules. Whatever your loved one's situation, it may be helpful to tailor exercise programs to individual preferences. You can help them do this. Finding ways to exercise together can also enhance your loved one's adherence to a routine and help nurture your relationship.

DIET

Diet is an important part of mental health. Some studies report associations between poor nutritional choices and mood symptoms (Li et al. 2017).

You can help your loved one make healthy dietary choices, as many people with SMI have poor diets and are unmotivated to cook. Financial limitations and location may limit some SMI patients' abilities to make healthy food choices. You can find dietary information at the MyPlate website of the US Department of Agriculture. You can also involve your loved one in meal planning to foster self-reliance and engagement. Finally, regular family meals can help facilitate healthy eating and strengthen relationships.

COMPLEMENTARY HEALTH

Certain nutritional, psychological, and physical interventions can complement traditional psychiatric treatment to help manage SMI symptoms. You can help your loved one by researching complementary approaches they or you are interested in, assessing both their positive and negative effects when combined with conventional medicine. For example, certain nutritional regimes might compromise medicine regimens and worse, they can potentially be dangerous.

Dismissing out of hand your loved one's interest in certain complementary approaches, like supplements or Eastern medicine, is often counterproductive. But encourage your loved one to consult with their psychiatrist or other doctor so they can make well-informed decisions about such approaches and optimize the results.

Finally, you might also join your loved one in relevant complementary activities, like yoga and meditation, which can reinforce their adoption and practice. Through these efforts, you can help promote a more comprehensive approach to wellness.

Intellectual Wellness

Intellectual wellness can involve many dimensions and practices that engage our brains and can expand our intellect, such as critical thinking, creativity, and other cerebral activities. You can foster intellectual wellness by encouraging your loved one to expand their knowledge and skills. There are a variety of options to develop these interests, such as online courses, reading, podcasts, hobbies, community and volunteer projects, and travel. These activities can benefit recovery. Certain complex mental activities (e.g., puzzle solving) are also a kind of exercise that can help foster cognitive function. And of course, these activities may offer opportunities to bond with your loved one.

Many people experience the onset of mental illness during their college years, with a significant proportion opting to discontinue their education. As previously mentioned, 75 percent of all lifetime mental illnesses emerge by the age of twenty-four, according to NAMI (n.d.). However, many people with SMI want to complete higher education, and many do.

If your loved one is in this situation, you're in a good position, as caregiver, to help them take proactive measures to cope with symptoms and manage academic demands. Your loved one can talk to advisors and professors about challenges and work with them to plan out an actionable curriculum and coursework. Online coursework may be an option that mitigates certain stresses. Your loved one may also take a partial course load to ease a potential burden, or take a formal medical leave, at points of acute stress, to facilitate a smoother potential return. Also consider accommodations they're entitled to under the ADA, such as extra time for assignments and exams.

Though resuming studies after a prolonged hiatus can pose challenges, people with SMI do successfully reengage with academic pursuits. It may be that feelings of shame or a sense of lagging behind peers who have graduated deter your loved one from considering a return to school if they previously took an absence. But pursuing further studies can serve as a powerful incentive for maintaining wellness, and it's crucial to consistently encourage your loved one in this regard.

Finally, supported education programs at community behavioral health centers and Clubhouses can help facilitate high school and college completion. These programs are tailored to the individual, considering their preferences, strengths, and unique experiences. As a supportive caregiver, you can actively contribute to your loved one's educational journey by assisting them in navigating these programs when applicable.

Environmental Wellness

The neighborhood's impact on mental health is significant. Good housing, access to public transportation, and availability of fresh food can positively influence mental health. Your ability to intervene on your loved one's behalf in these domains may be limited by your own circumstances. But there are resources to consider. Permanent supportive housing programs, coordinated by community behavioral health centers and Clubhouses, assist people with mental illness in securing safe, affordable housing.

For those in recovery from addiction, a sober living environment can be particularly beneficial. These aspects collectively constitute some of the social determinants of mental health (CDC 2024a).

Spiritual Wellness

Engaging in meditation, prayer, or other forms of spirituality can offer stress relief. Religion has been linked to enhanced remission in patients with depression. Some studies link a sense of spirituality and religious affiliation with enhanced resilience in the face of adversity and stress. Fostering a sense of spirituality, independent of any established religion, can also have mental health benefits. Further, spiritual wellness can provide your loved one with a sense of meaning and purpose in life. Encourage or jointly explore these pursuits with your loved one, if relevant, to foster this engagement.

Social Wellness

Staying connected with family and friends is crucial for managing stress. However, your loved one may experience family or friends as a possible source of stress. You might gently explore ways in which your loved one identifies support versus conflict in various relationships with friends and family. Encourage your loved one to reach out, too—to make new friends and participate in volunteer and community activities. Clubhouses like Fountain House serve as social clubs for people with SMI that also focus on achieving goals related to relationship building, wellness, education, and employment. They promote unity and belonging.

Peer support is a valuable resource. Peers share similar experiences, providing relatable perspectives. While engaging in the mental health community is essential, broadening social contacts is equally important for a well-rounded identity.

You can facilitate social engagement by learning about available options, participating in local activities, and organizing family events.

Exploring Change

Addressing triggers and promoting wellness often requires change. Be sensitive to your loved one's readiness for change. The Stages of Change model from chapter 3 may help you assess your loved one's readiness to make change. You can use gentle questions to encourage discussions about change and start planning specific changes and the process to achieve them. Goals should be tailored to your loved one's preferences and needs. The S.M.A.R.T. framework can be helpful (chapters 2 and 3).

You also play a much bigger role than you might think in helping your loved one rebuild motivation, optimism, and self-esteem, which are crucial for effective change. Praising accomplishments, no matter how small, is vital. Small steps build on each other, contributing to more significant achievements. Acknowledging and celebrating these accomplishments are integral to the recovery process.

Daily Wellness Plan

Turning self-care activities into habits and incorporating them into daily routines is crucial for effective self-care. You can help create a schedule of activities and engaging in them with your loved one. It may help to think of your role as being an "accountability buddy" and providing options rather than forcing activity.

EXERCISE: Creating a Behavioral Contract

A behavioral contract, as discussed earlier, is an evidence-based approach to motivate loved ones in their treatment plan. It involves rewarding agreed-upon actions, promoting positive behavior, and empowering the loved one.

To create a contract, you can start by answering these questions:

1. What realistic goals would you and your loved one like to set?

2. What achievable steps would your loved one like to take to achieve each goal?

3. What rewards will you and your loved one institute for achievement of the steps? And the goals?

4. What accountability mechanisms and mutual agreements do you want to set for your loved one—and which ones does your loved one wish to set for you?

Flexibility, consistency, and mutual involvement between you and your loved one in setting rewards is crucial to achieving the intended results.

Conclusion

Addressing SMI requires a holistic approach. Combining various wellness dimensions with strategies for change, goal setting, routine, and positive reinforcement contributes to overall wellness. Your role in providing support, understanding, and actively participating in various aspects of your loved one's life is paramount. Building a collaborative, respectful relationship will enhance the effectiveness of interventions. Recognizing achievements, fostering a sense of accomplishment, and creating an environment that supports the pursuit of a fulfilling and balanced life will be invaluable in your loved one's journey to recovery.

CHAPTER 8

Talking About Mental Illness

Talking about mental illness is the first step in getting support. But you shouldn't wait for your loved one to reach out to you. If they don't, you should "reach in" to them. Break through communication barriers created by stigma.

Effective communication with your loved one significantly impacts your relationship and your ability to support them. Good communication enhances trust and reduces misunderstandings, encouraging your loved one to be more open about their struggles and collaborate with their treatment team. Poor communication can lead to misunderstandings, disagreements, and relationship breakdowns, contributing to your loved one's withdrawal and isolation.

Talking about mental illness requires thoughtfulness but isn't as difficult as people may think. While there's no universal way to talk about mental illness, there are best practices that can help you initiate productive discussions over time. In this chapter, we'll guide you through various strategies for talking with your loved one about their SMI symptoms, treatment, and more. We will start with two communication fundamentals.

Key Communication Fundamentals

Fundamental 1: *Empathy*

Empathy, being sensitive to another person's experience, can unify your relationship with your loved one. Infusing your actions and communications with empathy can bring you closer. As a result, you many better understand your loved one's fears and hopes, enabling you to align your actions with shared goals for their recovery.

Teresa Wiseman (1996) summarizes the four basic attributes of empathy as

1. *See the world as others see it*

2. *Nonjudgmental*

3. *Understanding another's feelings*

4. *Communicate the understanding*

A simple rule of thumb for showing your loved one empathy is to treat them as a person, not an illness. For example, when your loved one expresses disappointment or pessimism, you could suggest that their illness might distort how they see themself in less favorable ways than you and others do. Too often the focus of SMI becomes the illness and not the person experiencing it.

People struggling with mental illness frequently also grapple with feelings of being profoundly misunderstood. Consequently, building your knowledge of mental illness can significantly elevate your effectiveness as a caregiver.

Fundamental 2: *Agency and Autonomy*

Helping your loved one regain agency and control over their actions is crucial. Mental illness can make them feel like they've lost control over their own existence. They might feel like they're unable to lead the life they desire, which is compounded when others attempt to control them.

So, you should know that, even though your intentions may be well-meaning, any attempts you make to dictate or take over aspects of your loved one's life can be profoundly distressing to them and counterproductive to their treatment. You may have reservations about their choices, but unless a given choice poses an imminent risk to the safety of your loved one or others, you should not get in the way. Often, we derive our most valuable insights from our own errors and misjudgments.

Structuring Conversations with Your Loved One

Initial conversations set the tone for future discussions. Overcoming a negative start to these conversations can be challenging. It can prove difficult to correct misunderstandings or negative impressions that may have been formed in initial dialogue. Subsequent conversations often become smoother and more constructive.

Talking about the mental illness itself can be very hard, particularly when you and your loved one don't have a professional understanding and insights. But you can talk about triggers and symptoms. Initiating discussions by focusing on specific triggers, like relationship challenges, can be effective. It can also help to discuss symptoms as responses, at least to some degree, to their environment and situations, not something that's particular to them or "wrong" with them. Focusing on triggers and symptoms can help normalize the experience of mental illness, mitigating the stigma and mystery that gets in the way of the discussion.

Find ways to relate more closely to your loved one's situation. This may involve sharing your own mental health experiences. In all your interactions, the most important principle for you to uphold is hope. Always exhibit a positive outlook and emphasize love and support. Continuously reinforce the idea that it's "we" together, not "you" alone, who will navigate through these challenges.

Consistently reassure your loved one that mental health recovery is attainable and validate their emotions. Always maintain a collaborative approach by asking your loved one "Can I assist you?" and "What can I do to support you?" rather than imposing your views or trying to set the arrangements you think are best. You want them to retain control over their situation.

Get Informed

Ensure you're educated about mental illness, including early warning signs, specific conditions, symptom treatment methods, and self-care practices. You should also understand both stigma and self-stigma to avoid making stigmatizing statements and address stereotypes that your loved one may be processing. If needed, seek guidance from a therapist or psychiatrist to better prepare for these conversations.

Also work to understand your loved one's experience, as best you can. Compile a mental or written list of any changes you've observed in your loved one's feelings, thoughts, and behaviors. Sharing these observations with your loved one in the conversation can also help you have more concrete and constructive discussions with them.

Objectives

For any productive conversation, it's also essential to establish clear objectives and define desired outcomes. Identify the most critical issues to address to help make the conversation focused and purposeful.

A key factor is to consider where your loved one is in their mental health journey. The Stages of Change framework discussed in chapter 3 can help you. Draw from the insights in that chapter to tailor your approach to align with your loved one's specific stage.

During the conversation, create space for your loved one to express their thoughts and feelings about the objective you've identified. Allow your loved one to express their reasons for either maintaining their current situation or embracing positive change.

Be attentive to any indications that your loved one may not be fully prepared for change. Often, this reluctance is revealed in statements that include the word "but." For example, they might say "I'd like to take my medication, but..." It's helpful to be ready with a balanced list of pros and cons, along with alternative actions, to address these objections. Present these suggestions gently and consider asking for permission before offering them. Employ phrases like "maybe," "I don't know," or "I know you know best" to express sensitivity to and respect for your loved one's views.

If your objective is to encourage your loved one to seek treatment, come prepared with relevant resources that can provide them with valuable information and options.

Participants

Involve family members in discussions and reach a collective view on what to address. Designate a discussion leader. When involving friends or family, be sensitive to what information you share so you do not violate your loved one's privacy.

Preparation

Prepare for conversations by outlining talking points and imagining potential reactions. Select a suitable time and place. Try to have the conversation when your loved one is feeling well and likelier to be more constructive. Choose a calm and relaxed setting to encourage openness and minimize adverse reactions. Focus on controlling your emotions and maintaining your composure. Have a contingency plan in the event your loved one becomes upset during the conversation.

Having the Actual Conversation

You might allow your loved one to take the lead in the talk by asking them what they would like to share or discuss. Be prepared for moments of silence; sometimes, simply listening and offering minimal responses like "aahaa" can be immensely helpful. Your loved one may not always seek a conversation but might find comfort in having someone who listens. If they want to talk, utilize the active listening techniques discussed below.

Focus on you loved one's body language, particularly negative cues that may signal a shift in tone. These cues include poor posture, avoiding eye contact, crossed arms, and fidgeting. Maintain emotional composure and adapt your communication style to match your loved one's temperament. Use concise language and straightforward sentences.

Address your implicit biases, as caregivers can unintentionally contribute to stigma. Recognize that your loved one may be highly sensitive to stigmatizing language and actions. Try to anticipate the impact of your response before answering. If you make a mistake, recognize it, and apologize for it.

If your loved one initially refuses to engage, gently encourage them. Should they remain reluctant, respect their privacy, and stop the discussion. Resist the urge to interrupt during the conversation. If a conversation has become too charged to be helpful, it can be useful to say "The things you're telling me are so important. Why don't we take a break to reflect and then come back to this later?"

Follow-Up

After each discussion, make a note of what works and doesn't work and adjust your approach, word choice, and more, the next time. Learn to adapt your communication according to the person's mood.

Give your loved one time to consider the discussion. Gently follow up.

When SMI Makes Communication Hard

Some symptoms can pose significant obstacles to effective communication. These may include difficulties with concentration, a pessimistic outlook on the future, extreme mood fluctuations, apathy, delusions, hallucinations, or other disruptions in thinking. When your loved one is grappling with such symptoms, they may have limited control over their actions. Be prepared to manage these situations. The de-escalation strategies discussed in chapter 3, Working with Your Loved One Effectively in Recovery, may be helpful.

Righting Reflex

You might find yourself wanting to "fix" your loved one. Caregivers, by instinct, often long to restore their loved one to health or help them attain what they see as optimal well-being. This inclination can bring out an appearance of authority, even if you're not consciously aware of it. This is referred to as the "righting reflex" (Rollnick, Miller, and Butler 2022).

However, it's important to understand that your loved one will often resist such attempts at persuasion. Research has shown that when we attempt to correct someone's behavior, they tend to resist change even more. Rosengren (2017) cautions against trying to convince someone that they have an issue, why or how to change, or the risks of not changing.

Be as honest as you can about what you're seeing and feeling, and what you think your loved one might be going through, to try to agree on what might need to change and how. If a particular aspect of your loved one's thinking or behavior concerns you, gently inquire whether they recognize the issue and have a desire to make changes. This will help you determine if you are both on the same page.

Communication Techniques

The way you communicate with your loved one can be as important as what you communicate. The following are communication techniques that may help you have more constructive discussions with your loved one.

OPEN-ENDED QUESTIONS

Avoid yes-or-no questions as they can feel like interrogations. Instead, use open-ended questions to encourage and sustain conversations. Responses can take the form of questions or statements to increase engagement between you and your loved one.

To ensure productive communication, avoid bombarding your loved one with questions. Instead, adopt a listening-oriented approach, limit your talking, and allow time for calm responses.

Here are some examples of open-ended questions:

- What are your reservations about medication?

- How did making that change in your daily routine make you feel?

- What do you think might help you take better care of yourself?

The following are typical ways to begin an open-ended question:

- How do you think you could benefit from...?

- How do you feel about...?

- What worries do you have about...?

- What can we do to help...?

- In what way could you...?

- What are your plans to...?

- What do you think you should do?

ACTIVE LISTENING

Active listening is giving your full attention to your loved one when they speak, considering their emotions, the environment, and their body language. You should maintain eye contact if it's a face-to-face conversation. This approach helps filter out distractions, understand incoming information, and respond thoughtfully. Active listening doesn't mean always agreeing with the information received. Instead, it prioritizes being a responsive and nonjudgmental listener.

Here are some tips for being an active listener:

- Show sensitivity to your loved one's thoughts and feelings
- Exhibit empathy by recalling your own struggles
- Refrain from interrupting and eliminate distractions
- Hold off on forming judgments until the message is fully conveyed
- Pay attention to body language
- Maintain an open-minded attitude
- Express genuine interest and attentiveness
- Seek clarification when necessary
- Offer meaningful feedback
- Summarize key points
- Be patient
- Stay fully engaged

Here are a few specific techniques to help you put these principles into practice:

Rephrase: Periodically rephrase what you believe your loved one has expressed—rather than simply repeating, put it into your own words. For instance, you can say "Let me make sure I've got this right..."

Unpack: Help your loved one better understand and acknowledge what they said. Suppose your loved one confides, "I'm worried I won't wake up in time..." You might respond, "It seems like you could use some help getting up?"

Confirm: Summarize the various details of the issue to confirm your understanding of the situation.

Explore: Encourage deeper insights with questions. For example, "What do you think would happen if you...?" Utilize leading questions to gather additional details, such as "Would you like to elaborate?", "What happened afterward?", and "Could you provide more background?"

Share: Share your thoughts on the situation with your loved one. Then, carefully listen to your loved one's reaction to confirm they understand it.

Affirm: Recognize your loved one's challenges, concerns, and emotions. Listen with empathy and an engaged response, like "I admire your willingness to discuss such a challenging issue..."

Deliver: Intentionally pause at moments to emphasize points and allow your loved one to take in your feedback. This signals to your loved one that you're conveying something of importance.

Space: Embrace comfortable silences that create space for a patient exchange. Give your loved one both time to contemplate and space to articulate their thoughts.

Redirect: Shift conversation topics or pause the discussion if your loved one exhibits signs of excessive aggression, agitation, or anger.

Assess: Explore the potential outcomes of inaction. Be sure to do so in a way that avoids the righting reflex discussed above.

COLLABORATIVE COMMUNICATION

Collaborative communication can begin with determining what stage of change (see chapter 3) your loved one is at. The following strategies can help you engage with your loved one and gain their acceptance to help as they try to make positive change.

Asking for permission. Empower your loved one by asking permission to help them. Consider asking permission to:

- Share information: "Would you like me to help you gather more information on your medications?"

- Explore your loved one's comments: "Would you like to talk more about that?"

- Discuss alternatives: "I know some options I have heard work for others. Would you like to hear about them?"

Asking permission allows your loved one to determine what to do. It gives them the freedom to choose what to discuss and share with you.

Affirmations. Validate your loved one's strengths and emotions. Focus on specific behaviors and successes: "I think you've done well. Consider the progress you've achieved. How does that make you feel?"

Or, if your loved one says something like "I moved my morning medication to the kitchen table, so I won't forget to take it with breakfast," you might respond with "That's a great idea. I hope it's effective."

Reframing. Reframing is a type of affirmation. When reframing, you transform a negative statement or experience into a positive. Reframing is a valuable tool for lessening your loved one's resistance. It can help you gently steer a conversation from a negative tone or context toward a more positive perspective and facilitate more constructive exploration of issues.

Here's an example of how to reframe a loved one's negative comment:

Loved one: "I've tried and failed so many times to get into a weekly exercise routine."

Caregiver: "You've displayed remarkable determination."

Confidence building. Confidence is important because taking action requires embracing certain risks. Your loved one may lack confidence. Self-stigmatization may convince your loved one that they're destined to fail and that their condition won't improve. You must provide unwavering support and encouragement, most importantly when they experience setbacks or face challenges.

Communicating respect and trust. Always honor your loved one's wishes. If they are adults, treat them as individuals capable of making their own choices. Even if they're minors, treat their desires and preferences as worthy of consideration. This is a demonstration of respect for them.

Trust should also be at the forefront of your communication. Building trust between you and your loved one is key for better treatment and life outcomes. For instance, if you wish to discuss matters with your loved one's healthcare provider, request your loved one's permission rather than contacting the doctor without their knowledge. If your loved one expresses objections, it's perfectly fine to inquire about their concerns, as this can help clarify trust-related issues. If they ask you not to share certain details, respect their wishes unless it poses a risk to their safety or that of others. If you can't respect their wishes for this reason, communicate that to them clearly and kindly as you can.

Maintaining honesty. Be sensitive but honest and direct about your concerns. Your loved one may benefit from hearing how their behaviors might hurt them—physically, socially, emotionally, professionally, and so forth—or how their behaviors affect you or others.

Difficult discussions can ultimately lead to significant breakthroughs. Following a tough discussion, provide your loved one with the opportunity to reflect on what was said. If the conversation leads to anger, don't automatically assume that your loved one is angry with you. It is more likely that they are frustrated with the situation itself.

Avoiding defensiveness. Use constructive phrasings to keep conversations open. The key principles are to convey to your loved one understanding, support, and a desire to collaborate rather than frustration over what you think they need to do. Recognize that your loved one may respond defensively because they feel the need to protect their own feelings.

Below are examples of communication blockers to be avoided and alternative, more constructive phrasings to keep conversations open:

Communication Blocker	Instead of Saying	Say This
Accusing	"You didn't take your meds."	"I respect that you manage your medication, but we both want to guard against the risk of relapse when you miss doses. How can we work on this together?"
Alarmed	"I think you're getting manic."	"I notice you're acting differently than your normal self. Would it be okay if we called your doctor together? I can share my perspective with you present."
Arguing	"I don't care what you think, this is my home."	"We live here together, and it's important that we agree on things."
Controlling	"You are going to take this medication."	"I can't control what you do but taking your medication may be helpful."
Criticizing	"I can't stand it when you..."	"Would it be possible to talk to you about..."
Generalizing	"You always..." or "You never..."	"Can we talk about when you..."

If you fall into defensive communication patterns, recognize it, apologize, and start again. Differences in tone can significantly impact your relationship and ability to work with your loved one.

Situations to Be Prepared For

You will want to prepare for potentially extreme situations that may arise from you loved one's SMI over time, including arguments, refusals of help, and suicidal behavior. Below we discuss strategies to address these situations.

Arguments

Resist being drawn into arguments with your loved one. When discussions become argumentative, shift the topic, or pause.

You may find yourself in this situation when your loved one behaves angrily toward you. Many caregivers think that their loved one is angry with them. But people with SMI often project their anger at their situation onto their caregivers. It's also common to become frustrated and angry when your loved one appears to act against their best interests. These situations can be highly sensitive for both you and your loved one. It's essential not to take these circumstances personally.

Establish clear boundaries to protect against abusive behavior. You might set expectations for the consequences of this type of treatment. You may have to distance yourself or others physically from your loved one or even call the police in the most extreme situations.

Refuses Help

Again, there can be many reasons why your loved one is reluctant to accept help or engage in communication about their mental illness, including stigma, fear of an uncertain future, lack of understanding or denial of their condition, and more.

Most of these can be mitigated through education. But while you can attempt to educate your loved one, they might question your knowledge, or think you're overreacting. In some cases, they might be more receptive to information from a friend, or someone less directly involved in the situation—perhaps even a mental health provider.

Nevertheless, you can still support your loved one. You can compile resources for them to read at their own pace. You can help find someone with whom they feel comfortable discussing their illness. You can offer your loved one an incentive, such as a gift or privilege, as part of a behavioral contract (discussed in chapter 7). Whatever your approach, always aim to encourage rather than coerce or pressure your loved one into seeking treatment. People with mental illness commonly need time to come to terms with the possibility of having a mental illness, so patience is key.

If your loved one refuses help, consider writing a heartfelt letter to them. Begin by acknowledging the challenges they're facing and express your pride in them. Share your concerns and reassure them that improvement is possible. Be nostalgic. Remind them of when things were better and assure them that they can feel that way again. Ask them if you can help. Let them know that you're willing to do whatever it takes to see them well and that you will always be there for them.

Suicidal Behavior

Talk openly about suicidal behavior, including ideation. Take all conversations about suicide seriously and never promise confidentiality. As previously mentioned, contrary to popular belief, "acknowledging and talking about suicide may reduce suicidal ideation and may lead to improvements in mental health in treatment-seeking populations" (Dazzi et al. 2014). There is a no guaranteed way to predict suicidal behavior. It is sometimes planned but is more often impulsive. It often correlates to severity of depression. Suicide risk is especially high in people who have made a previous attempt, especially with highly lethal methods. Importantly, if a loved one is experiencing suicidal thoughts, they may be very reluctant to share for fear of consequences such as hospitalization. If you are concerned that your loved may be suicidal, you could try to open up a conversation by saying something like "If you were having suicidal thoughts, would you be afraid to reveal them or would you trust that the response you get would be compassionate and collaborative."

Lacks Insight

As discussed in chapter 1, your loved one may lack insight, or be unaware, that they have a mental illness. This condition is called anosognosia.

One potential strategy for communicating with someone with anosognosia is LEAP, which stands for listen, empathize, agree, and partner. In essence, LEAP involves taking a nonjudgmental approach to communication that focuses on empathizing with how a loved one feels, finding common ground, and partnering to find solutions to problems, not judging whether their concerns are valid or accurate (Amador 2022).

Conclusion

In this chapter, we've reviewed various strategies for approaching and structuring conversations with loved ones, highlighting the core principles of empathy, agency, and autonomy. We introduced communication techniques such as open-ended questions, active listening, and collaborative communication and offered guidance on navigating potential challenges and sensitive situations you may encounter with your loved one. By adopting these approaches and maintaining honesty, respect, and trust in your interactions, you can create a supportive environment conducive to your loved one's recovery journey.

In the next chapter, we will focus on you—how to care for yourself while managing the challenges of being a caregiver to your loved one.

Caregiver Self-Care: For My Good and Their Good

CHAPTER 9

Most of this book focuses on how you, as a caregiver, can better support your loved one with SMI through the recovery journey. When you commit yourself to being a caregiver, you may find yourself immersed in this role, dedicating immense amounts of time and energy to protecting and helping your loved one. But this can't be your singular focus.

I (Izzy) am writing now to guide you, a caregiver to a person with SMI, to consider your own well-being on this journey toward your loved one's recovery. Prioritizing management of my wife's illness caused me to neglect my own well-being—physical, emotional, and social—for some time. This focus felt necessary; it was also, ultimately, counterproductive. It spawned negative emotions and behaviors that hurt me, my ability to help my loved one, and our relationship.

We need to recognize and attend to our own needs—as caregivers and people. When our families face the challenges of mental illness, our health and well-being are also put at risk. We must think of recovery as our journey, in which both we and our loved one overcome the challenges of mental illness to live fully. Caring for yourself will benefit both you and your loved one.

Mental Illness Martyr

It's natural to prioritize managing your loved one's condition when you're faced with the potentially disruptive and destructive effects of a SMI. I was propelled into this role after my wife's first manic episode and involuntary hospitalization. She would experience five manic episodes and three hospitalizations over eighteen years. In that time, I became her determined monitor and guardian.

The experience of hospitalization was very traumatic and disruptive to my wife. Years later, I recognized that I also experienced trauma from these events—trauma that went unaddressed for too long. It helps explain why I tried to do and control everything I could to protect against another crisis.

I championed my wife through lows and pushed her toward her potential. But I also felt held back at times by the attention I was focusing on my wife's wellness. I redirected my energies toward my wife's treatment of my own volition, out of love and care, but I also allowed feelings of duty and responsibility to color how I viewed my role.

The caregiver role increasingly defined me. The stress, fear, and unaddressed trauma took an emotional toll on me. These changes led to resentment of my wife, to distancing from friends and family due to the stigma, and to neglect of personal needs in order to hold the pieces of our life together.

And I showed it. I certainly developed a sense of self-pity. In fact, when we argued, my wife used to tell me to stop being a mental illness martyr. As much as I pushed back on that, I did feel somewhat unfairly punished and burdened by my caregiver role. Perhaps neglecting my own health was a way to make my martyrdom a reality.

With time, and persistent work toward wellness on both our parts, my spouse found hope and her path to recovery. As she took more responsibility, a crucial realization dawned on me: I needed to take more responsibility for my own care. I didn't want to be the martyr. Being a caregiver didn't and shouldn't define me; I should define it.

Caregiver Self-Care

Below I share some of my insights on caring for yourself as a caregiver. The discussion is organized into three parts. First, being a caregiver is a unique role that we are typically thrown into untrained. But there are healthy and constructive ways to think about it. We then discuss how to cope with common emotions and experiences as a caregiver. Finally, we talk about how to care for yourself to avoid a martyr mindset and optimize your own health. In embracing these components of self-care, I've discovered the strength that emerges when caregivers prioritize their well-being, creating a more resilient and supportive care relationship.

Defining Your Role as a Caregiver

In becoming a caregiver, you may feel like your life and your relationship with your loved one are transformed. You will have many mixed emotions. You may feel sympathy for your loved one. You may feel sorry for yourself. You may question why it happened to you. You may worry about the stigma, what people will think about you. You may wonder what you might've done to contribute to your loved one's illness. Your future may feel uncertain. You may feel a huge sense of responsibility to care for your loved one.

These feelings are all fair and understandable. Don't push them away. Accept and address them. Otherwise, they may threaten to weaken and weigh you down in the journey that follows.

Actively define your role as a caregiver, rather allowing the responsibilities of caring for your loved one to define you. You can and should have a constructive view of the caregiver experience. After all, you are not alone. So many are doing what you are. We know from their experience (and mine) that it is manageable. And while SMI will require adjustments and changes in your interaction with your loved one, it doesn't have to define you or your relationship.

Over time, I learned to view my role as caregiver more positively by recognizing the below principles. You may benefit from them too:

No longer shouldering all: Let go of the burden of feeling solely responsible for your loved one's health by embracing a collaborative approach. This may help ease the pressure you may feel (which might also lead to resentment toward your loved one). It also helps you recognize that mental health is a shared responsibility and leads you to involve your loved one in their own care. You not only lighten the emotional burden on yourself but also empower your loved one to actively participate in their recovery. This fosters your loved one's autonomy and encourages them to take responsibility for their well-being. Caregiving becomes a partnership. This supportive environment promotes a more sustainable and effective recovery.

Anticipating without fear: Shift from waiting for disaster to occur to recognizing the risks of future episodes and managing them. By embracing this approach, you transform fear and anticipation of crisis into proactive awareness of the challenges that may arise over time. You develop a strategic mindset, identifying potential triggers and early signs of relapse and preparing to address them prudently and effectively. Often, this not only improves your preparedness but also empowers you to guide your loved one in developing their own coping strategies. This shift from fear to proactive management can contribute significantly to the stability of your loved one's mental health and facilitate a smoother recovery journey.

Empowerment through knowledge: You'll benefit immensely from working to understand your loved one's condition, triggers, and symptom management. Educating yourself this way requires work, but if you're reading this, you're clearly willing to put in that work. This knowledge better equips you to understand your loved one's challenges, and to know when and how to provide informed support to meet your loved one's needs. Moreover, when you share this knowledge with your loved one, it enhances their self-awareness. An empowered caregiver, armed with knowledge, becomes an advocate for their loved one. Your efforts to learn and understand will contribute to better treatment outcomes and an improved quality of life for you and your loved one.

Collaborative approach: This principle emphasizes the importance of teamwork in the caregiving process. Develop a good working relationship with your loved one and their providers, which can prevent contentious power dynamics within this support team. Keep open lines of communication with your loved one and their providers. Your insights into your loved one's daily life can complement the medical perspective, improving treatment planning, ensuring that both emotional and medical aspects are addressed, and enhancing the overall effectiveness and holism of the care provided.

Healing from guilt: Guilt can be a heavy burden for caregivers, especially regarding decisions like hospitalizations. If you're struggling with guilt, acknowledge that certain actions had to be taken in the best interests of your loved one's health and safety. Recognize that the challenges of mental illness sometimes leave you with limited options to protect your loved one, yourself, and others. Recognize, too, the possibility of repair of mistakes you might make along the way. Letting go of unnecessary guilt allows you to be more present and supportive. This creates a more compassionate and understanding caregiving environment. It also enables you to focus on the present and future, contributing to a healthier and more optimistic atmosphere and relationship.

Advocate for policy changes: You might join advocacy groups to influence policy impacting your loved one and others with mental illness, as well as other caregivers. Taking a stand for policy changes demonstrates a commitment to the well-being not only of your loved one but also the broader population affected by mental health issues. Your advocacy can also extend beyond your personal caregiving journey, positively impacting the mental health landscape for the broader population and future generations.

How to Respond to Caregiving Challenges

We'll now explore how to respond to manage a range of common difficult experiences across the stages of caregiving. These insights should help you enhance your own well-being while improving the support you provide your loved one on the path to recovery.

NAVIGATING DIFFERENT STAGES

Initial symptoms or onset. Your loved one is experiencing some of the symptoms discussed in chapter 1 for the first time. They haven't yet sought help or treatment and may not appreciate that they have a condition.

Acknowledge the challenges posed to your loved one by these changes. Encourage open communication about their experiences, fears, and uncertainties. Reassure your loved one and encourage them to seek professional guidance to understand and address the symptoms.

Understand the complexities involved when your loved one might be resistant to seeking help. Approach the situation with empathy, recognizing your loved one's autonomy, but explore avenues for involuntary treatment if their actions appear to pose a danger to them or others.

Diagnosis. Your loved one has received a medical diagnosis and is still coming to terms with it.

Allow yourself and your loved one time to process and adapt. Recognize that a diagnosis is not a sentence—your old life will not die. Mental illness poses challenges, but there are actionable strategies to manage, cope, and overcome its difficulties.

Approach denial with empathy and patience, encouraging open discussions about the reality of the situation. Provide gentle guidance toward acceptance and seek professional support to navigate through your loved one's denial phase.

Seek support for yourself from mental health professionals, support groups, or therapists to navigate the emotional complexities associated with the diagnosis.

Conflict with your loved one. You and your loved one are having difficulty communicating about their condition and treatment. They might be resisting treatment. You might be pushing for them to address their condition or make other changes that you believe are in their best interests.

Refer to chapter 3 for strategies to manage conflicts and maintain a healthy and supportive connection with your loved one. Approach disagreements with empathy and understanding. Try to find common ground. Remember and remind your loved one that you are both fighting their illness and shouldn't be fighting each other. Mental health professionals can also provide more objective perspectives and help mediate care decisions.

Treatment. Try to actively participate in your loved one's treatment process. Strive for open communication about treatment decisions.

Educate yourself about any treatment plans and reinforce the opportunity they offer your loved one to get better. Be realistic too: treatment requires patience, makes its own demands on your loved one, and often involves trial and error and adjustment over time.

Hospitalization. Hospitalization may feel like the ultimate loss of control for your loved one. You'll both need to accept that you cannot control certain situations created by your loved one's illness. But these situations and limitations are temporary. You may both take some relief in the fact that hospitalization may have saved your loved one from an escalation of their episode and worse outcomes. The hospitalization may also serve as a catalyst for those changes, proving to your loved one and you that you both need to make certain changes.

Focus on providing emotional support to your loved one in this vulnerable time. You should also acknowledge and validate your own emotions and potential trauma from the hospitalization and circumstances leading to it. Seek support from friends, family, or mental health professionals to process any feelings of anxiety, guilt, or helplessness. Finally, embrace any opportunity to make positive changes prompted by the hospitalization.

Relapse. Approach relapses with a collaborative mindset. Encourage your loved one to include you in their treatment planning to help come back from relapse quicker. You should work closely with your loved one and their mental health professionals to adjust treatment plans.

Treat the relapse like a new learning experience. Analyzing triggers and other factors that contributed to the relapse can offer both you and your loved one a sense of control and understanding. You might identify new potential triggers or learn to better weigh known triggers, improving your ability to navigate future situations.

UNDERSTANDING AND RESPONDING TO YOUR EMOTIONS

We'll now discuss common emotional reactions you should expect to have as a caregiver and ways to respond to these emotions constructively.

Afraid—Identify and communicate your fears related to caregiving, working with your mental health professionals to develop coping strategies to alleviate anxiety. Be open with your loved one about shared fears and concerns.

Alienated—Connect with support groups of caregivers who share similar experiences. Foster relationships with friends and family who understand and support your caregiving role. Combat feelings of isolation through open communication.

Angry—Channel anger into constructive outlets. Practice mindfulness and communication techniques to express anger effectively. Seek professional guidance to explore the underlying causes of anger and develop coping strategies.

Burdened—Again, initiate open conversations with your loved one about the challenges and responsibilities you face as a caregiver. Share your feelings and collaborate on strategies to distribute responsibilities more effectively.

Grieved—Recognize caregiving as a journey of highs and lows, allowing yourself to grieve the losses, changes, and challenges in your life. Seek support from mental health professionals and support groups to navigate the grieving process. Engage in activities that support emotional healing for any losses experienced in the caregiving journey.

Guilty—Cultivate self-compassion and recognize the limits of control in caregiving. Embrace the idea that making decisions in the best interest of your loved one, even if difficult, is an act of love. These actions are guiltless. Shut down any thought that you contributed to or caused your loved one's condition. People do not cause mental illness. You are the opposite of the cause. You are a key part of the recovery.

Helpless—Develop a toolkit of coping strategies for moments of helplessness—seeking support from mental health professionals, engaging in self-care activities, and recognizing the aspects within your control.

Hopeless—Address such feelings through collaborative goal-setting and planning, engaging in activities that bring a sense of purpose and achievement to your loved one and you. Seek professional guidance through periods of despair.

Irritated—It's important to condition yourself to separate your loved one from their illness. In doing so, you can address your loved one's specific behaviors without negatively impacting your relationship. Channel feelings of irritation into constructive outlets and engage in self-reflection to understand the source of irritation and explore healthy coping mechanisms.

Resentful—Acknowledge feelings of resentment you may feel toward your loved one and explore their roots. Collaborate with your loved one to address underlying causes of resentment. This feeling may come as a surprise to your loved one, so it's helpful to put it on the table. Otherwise, your resentment may simmer and ultimately escalate without being checked.

Shaken—Acknowledge and accept the intense emotions that accompany mental health crises. Allow yourself space to process shock and chaos while maintaining a focus on practical solutions and emotional support for your loved one.

Traumatized—Acknowledge the potential for trauma in the care-giving journey. Seek therapeutic support to process trauma and develop resilience. Communicate openly with your loved one about shared experiences to foster understanding.

Underappreciated—Seek validation for your role as a caregiver and communicate your needs and feelings to your loved one. Fostering a mutual understanding and appreciation for caregiving responsibilities can help alleviate feelings of being underappreciated.

Finally, here are two positive qualities to foster.

Acceptance—Recognize that accepting your loved one's condition and your role as a caregiver are dynamic processes. Allow both yourself and your loved one the time and space to navigate through the stages of acceptance. Seek professional guidance as you need to.

Understanding—Foster an environment of empathy and understanding by communicating openly with your loved one about their experiences and emotions. Educate yourself about their mental health condition to enhance empathy and promote mutual support.

Caring for Yourself: Nurturing Your Well-Being as a Caregiver

Most of what we've discussed in this chapter is about better integrating your own needs as you interact with your loved one and address challenges created by their mental illness. This section offers strategies to improve and maintain your health while promoting your loved one's well-being.

As caregivers, we often feel guilt for prioritizing our own needs. It's crucial to acknowledge that engaging in self-care is not selfish. It's necessary for your overall well-being. You are a person with your own needs and interests which you deserve to have met. Being a caregiver doesn't change that. It doesn't make your health and well-being secondary to that of your loved one. Release yourself from the burden of guilt and embrace self-care as a guilt-free endeavor.

Disciplined focus on your own needs can help you counter feelings of resentment and burden that often arise as a caregiver and fight the isolation that the demands and even stigma from caring for your loved one may have created. In this way, establishing boundaries to prevent caregiving from defining you can help you break free from the constraints that you may have allowed caregiving to impose on you. This mindset will also make you a better caregiver because it may avoid or limit potential resentment toward your loved one that may manifest in nonconstructive interactions.

Caregiver burnout and fatigue. Acknowledging the prevalence of burnout and fatigue among caregivers is the first step toward addressing these issues. Grant yourself permission to feel and acknowledge your emotions. It's essential to recognize that sacrificing your own health and well-being for your loved one's care is unsustainable. You're an individual with your own needs and identity, separate from your caregiving roles.

Remember also that you don't need to be alone as a caregiver. You may have other family members and friends who can form part of your loved one's support network, helping with all kinds of tasks and situations that might ease the burden on you and enrich support for your loved one. These activities might be as seemingly mundane as household chores to help getting to doctor's appointments or spending time with your loved one. You should reach out to other people who can help.

Coping mechanisms. Prioritizing your physical and mental well-being is paramount. Consider the activities that promote your health and wellness as being as important as caring for your loved one's needs. Creating space for yourself, whether through mental health timeouts or personal activities, is essential for replenishing your energy and maintaining balance.

For me, establishing a workout regime was very valuable. And exercise doesn't have to be intensive. The structure and self-focused care it offers can benefit both physical and emotional health. It also offers an opportunity to engage with other people in a shared interest and familiar environment.

Establishing boundaries. Establishing clear boundaries is essential for maintaining your well-being as a caregiver. Communicate your needs and limits to your loved one. And prioritize your own space and time for rest, recharge, and socializing. This way, you can prevent burnout and maintain a healthy balance in your life.

I also reconnected with friends with whom I had fallen out of touch. In fact, one of my best friends and I started meeting for dinner every couple of months. I was able to speak openly with this person I trusted about whatever was on my mind—not just my wife's mental health. This was one of my best forms of therapy; it gave me something regular to look forward to.

Therapy. When your loved one has a SMI, it may feel like your own emotional challenges pale in comparison, and you may be inclined to put them aside. I did this for some time. I thought, *How can I see a psychiatrist when* *my wife's care is so much more serious?* But you must recognize that your loved one's condition exposes you to significant challenges, stresses, and even traumatic experiences. You cannot let these issues sit unaddressed, because they won't just sit there; they'll build on themselves and reveal themselves in negative ways.

Seeking therapy to address the emotional demands of caregiving can be immensely beneficial. Therapists can provide perspective on your range of feelings and offer strategies to cope with them effectively. Therapy offers a safe space to process your emotions and develop resilience in the face of caregiving challenges. Ongoing discussions with a therapist or psychiatrist can also help you gain insights and learn more about your loved one's condition and formulate strategies to address situations that might arise.

Therapy has been a key outlet and form of self-care for me. It reduced the isolation I felt as a caregiver. It also helped me better understand and, in turn, gain some command of my wife's condition and recovery journey. It helped validate and prioritize my own feelings and stresses through this process.

Family peer support. Family peer support has emerged as a valuable resource for people caring for loved ones with mental and physical illnesses. Various research studies highlight the effectiveness of family peer support interventions. For example, studies focusing on emerging mental health challenges found that family peer support enhanced knowledge about psychosis, coping strategies, and emotional support (Levasseur et al. 2019). Furthermore, interventions like the NAMI Family-to-Family Education Program have reported improvements in empowerment, knowledge, and self-care strategies among family members (Dixon et al. 2001). "Sharing first-person experiences is critical to NAMI's work and mission" (Duckworth 2022). By offering emotional support, guidance, and empowerment, family peer support interventions contribute to the well-being of both caregivers and their loved ones.

You may benefit from the support programs and resources offered by various organizations. NAMI, the largest grassroots mental health organization in the US, advocates for families with mental illness and provides free mental health programs and support services through its nationwide network of affiliate organizations. For instance, NAMI-NYC, one of its largest affiliates and serving the New York City area, offers peer-led classes, support groups, and a direct helpline for family members caring for loved ones with mental health challenges.

Additionally, the National Federation of Families (NFF) advocates for families with mental health and substance use challenges, offering a range of services through its affiliate family-run organizations. Other organizations, such as Mental Health America and the Depression and Bipolar Support Alliance, also offer valuable resources and support for caregivers in the mental health community. See a list of additional peer support resources at the end of this book.

Peer support can be particularly useful for caregivers navigating the dynamics and challenges of dual mental illness, where both the caregiver and their loved one have mental health conditions. If this describes your case, engaging with peers who share similar experiences can provide invaluable insights and support in managing the complexities of caregiving while also caring for your own mental health.

Conclusion

In conclusion, as a caregiver, it's critical to prioritize your own well-being while supporting your loved one with mental illness. Neglecting your own health and needs may undermine your ability to provide effective care and support. In this chapter, you learned key strategies to nurture your own well-being by:

- Defining your role as a caregiver and adopting a constructive view of the caregiving experience

- Acknowledging and addressing common emotions experienced by caregivers, such as irritation, underappreciation, and fear

- Establishing boundaries, implementing coping mechanisms, seeking therapy, and accessing peer support

Incorporating these strategies into your life as a caregiver enables you to navigate the challenges of caregiving more effectively while fostering resilience and well-being for yourself and your loved one. You'll not only enhance your ability to provide support but also create a more compassionate and supportive caregiving environment overall.

Acknowledgments

I have many incredible supporters to thank for helping me reach and live in recovery and enabling me to help others do the same.

But only one person traveled that entire journey with me. When my struggles were greatest, I had only him. It was really hard at times, but love is greater than any mental illness. My spouse, my Izzy, helped me get here and keeps me here. He is a part of everything I do. He allows me to live a life of helping others.

I have several others to thank, most especially my loving parents, Maria and Carlos, for showing me the power of faith; Dude, my beloved cat, who never left my side in the depths of my depression; Max, my beloved Frenchie, who was with me in the early days of recovery and brought so much joy into my home; Chaya Weinstein, my kind occupational therapist, who first connected me with my peers; Joseph Goldberg, my amazing psychiatrist, whose treatment guided me to recovery; and Larry Davidson, my wonderful mentor, who made me truly realize the value of my lived experience.

I am also grateful to Mel, my cat and constant companion; Jane Thompson and Paul Kleindorfer, formerly of the Wharton School, whose compassionate support helped me complete my MBA; Nuno de Sousa Pereira, my only friend at Wharton, whose genuine care helped me stick it out through the early days of my illness; Fabiola Costa Girao, who made me realize that there is more to live for and gave me perspective at my lows; my ForLikeMinds community, which has supported my efforts to create a network of peers that empower each other; my NAMI-NYC family, especially Nathan Romano and Matt Kudish, who embraced and nurtured me in the early days of my recovery; my Yale PRCH family, especially Chyrell Bellamy and Annie Harper, who are examples of caring academics who thoughtfully incorporate people living with mental illness into their work to achieve the best outcomes; and my many, many Psych Ward Greeting Cards collaborators, especially Lisa DeFelice-Fratto and Barb Murak, who have strongly supported my mission to help members of our community when their struggles may be greatest. And I have so many more to thank for supporting my recovery and my work.

Finally, I am thankful for the one in twenty-five living with SMI, especially peer support specialists, for your courage and strength to fight for recovery and inspire so many like me.

—Katherine

I would like to acknowledge so many people, unnamed here, who have opened up and shared with me their own experiences as families with mental illness. They have allowed me to shake the feelings of isolation and stigmatization that too often burden families with mental illness. When they connected with me as someone with the common bond of mental illness, they also provided me with support. Their openness and courage have strengthened and motivated me to help other families impacted by mental illness. Finally, I have been inspired by Katherine's courage and resilience to do more when made to feel less. Her almost self-willed recovery has shown me what is possible with grit and determination—and a little support.

—Izzy

This book would not have been possible without Jed Bickman, our wonderful acquisitions editor at New Harbinger, who believed our story could help others, and the editorial expertise of Vicraj Gill. We are tremendously grateful for this opportunity.

US Resources

There are many mental health resources. You might find this list helpful.

Crisis and Emergency

988 Suicide and Crisis Lifeline call, text, chat

911 Emergency call or text

988 and 911: Please note the similarities and differences (The National Council for Mental Wellbeing)

988 Suicide and Crisis Lifeline, Spanish call 988, press 2, text AYUDA to 988

Crisis Text Line, text HOME to 741741

Local Mobile Crisis services

Disaster Distress Helpline, 1-800-985-5990

Trevor Project (for LGBTQ+ youth), 1-866-488-7386, text 678678

US Veterans Crisis Line, Dial 988 then press 1, text 838255

Warmlines

Warmlines are peer-run phone lines that provide emotional support by peers in recovery. You can obtain local contact information by calling your local NAMI helpline or online at https://www.warmline.org.

Helplines

Several mental health nonprofit organizations have helplines that can provide helpful information and referrals.

One of the best known is the NAMI helpline.
Call 1-800-950-NAMI (6264), text "Helpline" to 62640.

Many NAMI affiliates also have their own local helpline.

Reputable Online Sources

In addition to the above resources and your healthcare provider, there are many reputable online sources of information that may be helpful, which are listed below. Always confirm what you learn from these sources with your healthcare provider before acting on it.

American Academy of Child and Adolescent Psychiatry

American Psychiatric Association

American Psychological Association

Centers for Disease Control and Prevention

Cleveland Clinic

Department of Veterans Affairs

Mayo Clinic

National Institute of Mental Health

National Institute on Drug Abuse

National Library of Medicine—MedlinePlus (multiple languages)

Substance Abuse and Mental Health Administration—SAMHSA

Academic Research

Google Scholar

Medline

PubMed

Nonprofit organizations

Nonprofits organizations can be a good source of information and support. The list below includes well-known US national nonprofits who have local affiliates or otherwise offer services nationally. In addition to these, it may be very helpful to identify other local mental health resources. You may be able to obtain more information about these from your local library, religious organizations, educational institutions, or community behavioral health centers. Helplines offered by nonprofits may also be able to provide referrals.

Active Minds

Al-Anon

Alcoholics Anonymous

American Foundation for Suicide Prevention

Anxiety and Depression Association of America

Bazelon Center for Mental Health Law

Black Emotional and Mental Health Collective

Brain and Behavior Research Foundation

Bring Change to Mind

Caregiver Action Network

Carter Center

Center for Native American Youth

Child Mind Institute

Clubhouse International

CURESZ Foundation

Depression and Bipolar Support Alliance and +150 chapters

Dual Recovery Anonymous

Emotions Matter

Families for Depression Awareness

Fountain House

GAINS Center for Behavioral
Health and Justice
Transformation

Hearing Voices Network

Henry Amador Center
on Anosognosia

Indian Health Service

International OCD
Foundation

inseparable

JED Foundation

Jewish Together

Kennedy Forum

Letters to Strangers

Live Through This

Make the Connection

Mental Health America and
its nationwide network of
240 affiliates

Mental Health Association
for Chinese Communities

Mental Health Coalition

Nar-Anon

Narcotics Anonymous

National Alliance
on Caregiving

National Alliance on Mental
Illness (NAMI) and over 650 state
and local affiliate organizations
and highly informative guide,
"You Are Not Alone"
by K. Duckworth

National Asian American
Pacific Islander Mental Health
Association

National Association for Peer
Supporters

National Association of
State Mental Health Program
Directors

National Council for Mental
Wellbeing

National Eating Disorders
Association

National Education Alliance
for Borderline Personality
Disorder

National Empowerment
Center

National Guardianship
Association

National Federation of Families
(NFF) and approximately
115 affiliate organizations and its
very helpful SAMHSA-funded
National Family Support
Technical Assistance Center

National Guardianship Association

National Latino Behavioral Health Association

National Mental Health Consumers' Self-Help Clearinghouse

National Resource Center for Psychiatric Advanced Directives

One Mind

PFLAG and over 400 local chapters

Psych Ward Greeting Cards

Schizophrenia and Psychosis Action Alliance

Seize the Awkward

Shatterproof

SMART Recovery

Steve Fund

Suicide Awareness Voices of Education

This is My Brave

Trans Lifeline

Treatment Advocacy Center

Trevor Project

Vibrant Emotional Health

The mention of specific resources herein is for education purposes only and does not imply endorsement. We encourage you to carefully research each resource before use.

References

Alzahrani, N. 2021. "The Effect of Hospitalization on Patients' Emotional and Psychological Well-Being Among Adult Patients: An Integrative Review." *Applied Nursing Research* 61: 151488.

Amador, X. 2022. *I Am Not Sick I Don't Need Help!: How to Help Someone Accept Treatment*, 20th anni. ed. Peconic, NY: Vida Press.

American Institute of Stress. n.d. "Holmes-Rahe Stress Inventory." Last accessed May 28, 2024. https://www.stress.org/holmes-rahe-stress-inventory.

Angst, F., H. H. Stassen, P. J. Clayton, and J. Angst. 2002. "Mortality of Patients with Mood Disorders: Follow-Up over 34–38 Years." *Journal of Affective Disorders* 68(2–3): 167–81.

Anthony, W. A. 1993. "Recovery from Mental Illness: The Guiding Vision of the Mental Health System in the 1990s." *Psychosocial Rehabilitation Journal* 16(4): 11–23.

Beck, A. T., G. Brown, and R. A. Steer. 1989. "Prediction of Eventual Suicide in Psychiatric Inpatients by Clinical Ratings of Hopelessness." *Journal of Consulting and Clinical Psychology* 57(2): 309–10.

Beck, J. S. 2020. *Cognitive Behavior Therapy: Basics and Beyond*, 3rd ed. New York: Guilford Press.

Bellamy, C., T. Schmutte, and L. Davidson. 2017. "An Update on the Growing Evidence Base for Peer Support." *Mental Health and Social Inclusion* 21(3): 161–67.

Centers for Disease Control (CDC). 2024a. "Social Determinants of Health (SDOH)." https://www.cdc.gov/about/priorities/why-is-addressing-sdoh -important.html.

———. 2024b. "Adverse Childhood Experiences (ACEs)." https://www.cdc .gov/aces/about/index.html.

Columbia University Department of Psychiatry. 2019. "Delusions May Stem from Sticky Beliefs, Study Finds." Columbia University Irving Medical Center, March 21. https://www.columbiapsychiatry.org/news/delusions -may-stem-sticky-beliefs-study-finds.

Corrigan, P. 2004. "How Stigma Interferes with Mental Health Care." *American Psychologist* 59(7): 614–25.

Corrigan, P., and D. Rao. 2012. "On the Self-Stigma of Mental Illness: Stages, Disclosure, and Strategies for Change." *The Canadian Journal of Psychiatry* 57(8): 464–69.

Croft, B., and N. Isvan. 2015. "Impact of the 2nd Story Peer Respite Program on Use of Inpatient and Emergency Services." *Psychiatric Services* 66(6): 632–37.

Davidson, L. and D. Roe. 2009. "Recovery from Versus Recovery in Serious Mental Illness: One Strategy for Lessening Confusion Plaguing Recovery." *Journal of Mental Health* 16(4): 459–70.

Davidson, L, D. Roe, and J. Tondora. 2020. "Concept and Model of Recovery." In *Schizophrenia Treatment Outcomes: An Evidence-Based Approach to Recovery*, edited by A. Shrivastava and A. De Sousa, 57–70. Cham: Springer Nature Switzerland AG.

Davidson, L., J. Tondora, M. S. Lawless, M. J. O'Connell, and M. Rowe. 2008. *A Practical Guide to Recovery-Oriented Practice*. Oxford: Oxford University Press.

Dazzi, T., R. Gribble, S. Wessely, and N. T. Fear. 2014. "Does Asking About Suicide and Related Behaviours Induce Suicidal Ideation? What Is the Evidence?" Psychological Medicine 44(16): 3361–63.

Dixon, L., B. Stewart, J. Burland, J. Delahanty, A. Lucksted, and M. Hoffman. 2001. "Pilot Study of the Effectiveness of the Family-to-Family Education Program." *Psychiatric Services* 52(7): 965–67.

Drucker, P. F. 1954. *The Practice of Management*. New York: HarperCollins.

Duckworth, K. 2022. *You Are Not Alone: The NAMI Guide to Navigating Mental Health with Advice from Experts and Wisdom from Real People and Families*. New York: Zando.

Elowe, J., J. Vallet, E. Castelao, M. F. Strippoli, M. Gholam, S. Ranjbar, J. Glaus, et al. 2022. "Psychotic Features, Particularly Mood Incongruence, as a Hallmark of Severity of Bipolar I Disorder." *International Journal of Bipolar Disorders* 10(1): 31.

Fiorillo, A., S. Barlati, A. Bellomo, G. Corrivetti, G. Nicolo, G. Sampogna, V. Stanga, et al. 2020. "The Role of Shared Decision-Making in Improving Adherence to Pharmacological Treatments in Patients with Schizophrenia: A Clinical Review." *Annals of General Psychiatry* 19: 43.

First, M. B. 2022. "Treatment of Mental Illness." *Merck Manual*. https://www.merckmanuals.com/home/mental-health-disorders/overview-of-mental-health-care/treatment-of-mental-illness.

Ghaemi, S. N., A. L. Stoll, and H. G. Pope Jr. 1995. "Lack of Insight in Bipolar Disorder. The Acute Manic Episode." *The Journal of Nervous and Mental Disease* 183(7): 464–67.

Goldberg, J. F., R. H. Perlis, C. L. Bowden, M. E. Thase, D. J. Miklowitz, L. B. Marangell, J. R. Calabrese, et al. 2009. "Manic Symptoms During Depressive Episodes in 1,380 Patients with Bipolar Disorder: Findings from the STEP-BD." *The American Journal of Psychiatry* 166(2): 173–81.

Holmes, T. H., and R. H. Rahe. 1967. "The Social Readjustment Rating Scale." *Journal of Psychosomatic Research* 11: 213–18.

Kendler, K., L. Karlowski, and C. Prescott. 1999. "Causal Relationship Between Stressful Life Events and the Onset of Major Depression." *The American Journal of Psychiatry* 156(6): 837–41.

Koenders, M. A., E. J. Giltay, A. T. Spijker, E. Hoencamp, P. Spinhoven, and B. M. Elzinga. 2014. "Stressful Life Events in Bipolar I and II Disorder: Cause or Consequence of Mood Symptoms?" *Journal of Affective Disorders* 161: 55–64.

Lazarus, R. S., and S. Folkman. 1984. *Stress, Appraisal, and Coping.* New York: Springer.

Lecomte, T., S. Potvin, C. Samson, A. Francoeur, C. Hache-Labelle, S. Gagne, J. Boucher, et al. 2019. "Predicting and Preventing Symptom Onset and Relapse in Schizophrenia—A Metareview of Current Empirical Evidence." *Journal of Abnormal Psychology* 128(8): 840–54.

Levasseur, M. A., M. Ferrari, S. McIlwaine, and S. N. Iyer. 2019. "Peer-Driven Family Support Services in the Context of First-Episode Psychosis: Participant Perceptions from a Canadian Early Intervention Programme." *Early Intervention in Psychiatry* 13(2): 335–41.

Li, Y., M.-R. Lv, Y.-J. Wei, L. Sun, J.-X. Zhang, H.-G. Zhang, and B. Li. 2017. "Dietary Patterns and Depression Risk: A Meta-Analysis." Psychiatry Research 253: 373–82.

Luciano, A., and E. Meara. 2014. "Employment Status of People with Mental Illness: National Survey Data from 2009 and 2010." *Psychiatric Services* 65(10): 1201–09.

McKay, M., J. C. Wood, and J. Brantley. 2019. *The Dialectical Behavior Therapy Skills Workbook: Practical DBT Exercises for Learning Mindfulness, Interpersonal Effectiveness, Emotion Regulation, and Distress Tolerance,* 2nd ed. Oakland, CA: New Harbinger Publications.

McLaughlin, C. 2004. "Delays in Treatment for Mental Disorders and Health Insurance Coverage." *Health Services Research* 39(2): 221–24.

Mental Health America (MHA). n.d. "Take a Mental Health Test." Last accessed May 28, 2024. https://screening.mhanational.org/screening-tools.

National Alliance on Mental Illness (NAMI). n.d. "Mental Health by the Numbers." Last accessed May 28, 2024. https://www.nami.org/about-mental-illness/mental-health-by-the-numbers.

———. n.d. "Mental Health Conditions." Last accessed May 28, 2024. https://www.nami.org/About-Mental-Illness/Mental-Health-Conditions.

———. n.d. "Schizophrenia." Last accessed May 28, 2024. https://www.nami.org/About-Mental-Illness/Mental-Health-Conditions/Schizophrenia.

National Alliance for Caregiving. 2016. "On Pins & Needles: Caregivers of Adults with Mental Illness." Presentation at the NAMI National Convention, Denver, CO, July 8.

National Association of State Mental Health Program Directors (NASMHPD) Medical Directors Council. 2006. *Morbidity and Mortality in People with Serious Mental Illness*. Alexandria, VA: NASMHPD.

National Council for Mental Wellbeing. n.d. "988 and 911: Similarities and Differences." Last accessed May 28, 2024. https://www.thenationalcouncil.org/988-and-911.

National Resource Center on Psychiatric Advance Directives. n.d. Last accessed May 28, 2024. https://nrc-pad.org.

National Institute of Mental Health (NIMH). n.d. "Bipolar Disorder." Last accessed May 28, 2024. https://www.nimh.nih.gov/health/statistics/bipolar-disorder.

———. n.d. "Major Depression." Last accessed May 28, 2024. https://www.nimh.nih.gov/health /statistics/major-depression.

———. n.d. "Mental Illness." Last accessed May 28, 2024. https://www.nimh.nih.gov/health/statistics/mental-illness.

———. n.d. "Suicide Prevention." Last accessed May 28, 2024. https://www.nimh.nih.gov/health/topics/suicide-prevention.

———. n.d. "Understanding Psychosis." Last accessed May 28, 2024. https://www.nimh.nih.gov/health/publications/understanding-psychosis.

Prochaska, J. O., and C. C. DiClemente. 1982. "Transtheoretical Therapy: Toward a More Integrative Model of Change." *Psychotherapy Theory, Research and Practice* 19(3): 276–88.

Ritsher, J. B., P. G. Otilingam, and M. Grajales. 2003. "Internalized Stigma of Mental Illness: Psychometric Properties of a New Measure." Psychiatry Research 121(1): 31–49.

Rollnick, S., W. R. Miller, and C. C. Butler. 2022. *Motivational Interviewing in Health Care: Helping Patients Change*. New York: Guilford Press.

Rosengren, D. B. 2017. *Building Motivational Interviewing Skills: A Practitioner Workbook*, 2nd ed. New York: Guilford Press.

Ruggero, C., R. Kotov, G. A. Carlson, M. Tanenberg-Karant, D. A. Gonzalez, and E. J. Bromet. 2011. "Consistency of the Diagnosis of Major Depression with Psychosis Across 10 Years." *Journal of Clinical Psychiatry* 72(9): 1207–13.

Substance Abuse and Mental Health Services Administration (SAMHSA). 2012. "SAMHSA's Working Definition of Recovery: 10 Guiding Principles of Recovery." https://store.samhsa.gov/product/samhsas-working-definition -recovery/pep12-recdef.

———. 2021. "National Survey on Drug Use and Health." Last accessed May 28, 2024. https://www.samhsa.gov/data/data-we-collect/nsduh -national-survey-drug-use-and-health.

———. 2023. "Key Substance Use and Mental Health Indicators in the United States: Results from the 2022 National Survey on Drug Use and Health." https://www.samhsa.gov/data/report/2022-nsduh-annual-national-report.

Slade, M. 2009. *Personal Recovery and Mental Illness: A Guide for Mental Health Professionals* (*Values-Based Practice*), 1st ed. Cambridge: Cambridge University Press.

Swarbrick, M. 2012. "A Wellness Approach to Mental Health Recovery in Recovery." In *People with Mental Illness: Philosophical and Related Perspectives*, edited by A. Rudnick, 30–38. Oxford: Oxford University Press.

Tedeschi, R., and L. G. Calhoun. 2004. "Target Article: 'Posttraumatic Growth: Conceptual Foundations and Empirical Evidence.'" *Psychological Inquiry* 15: 1–18.

Urits, I., K. Gress, K. Charipova, N. Li, A. Berger, E. M. Cornett, J. Hasoon, et al. 2020. "Cannabis Use and its Association with Psychological Disorders." *Psychopharmacology Bulletin* 50(2): 56–57.

Wiseman, T. 1996. "A Concept Analysis of Empathy." *Journal of Advanced Nursing* 23(6): 1162–67.

Wood, L., K. Martin, H. Christian, A. Nathan, C. Lauritsen, S. Houghton, I. Kawachi, et al. 2015. "The Pet Factor—Companion Animals as a Conduit for Getting to Know People, Friendship Formation and Social Support." *PLOS ONE* 10(4): e0122085.

Zubin, J., and B. Spring. 1977. "Vulnerability: A New View of Schizophrenia." *Journal of Abnormal Psychology* 86(2): 103–26.

Katherine Ponte is a mental health advocate, author, nonprofit leader, entrepreneur, coach, and lawyer. She is a certified psychiatric rehabilitation practitioner, and faculty member in the department of psychiatry's Program for Recovery and Community Health at Yale University. She built the ForLikeMinds platform of recovery-focused mental health initiatives and its associated community of over 100,000 that has reached millions. She is on the board of the National Alliance on Mental Illness-NYC. Katherine is author of *ForLikeMinds*. She has lived with severe bipolar I disorder with psychosis, including extended periods of suicidal depression for over twenty years, and has been happily living in recovery since 2018. She is based in New York, NY, and the Catskills.

Izzy Goncalves has worked in finance for nearly thirty years, and has been the primary caregiver for his spouse, Katherine. He has been instrumental in helping her develop several mental illness recovery initiatives. He is a *magna cum laude* and Phi Beta Kappa graduate from Brown University.

Foreword writer **Matt Kudish, LMSW, MPA**, is CEO of the National Alliance on Mental Illness of New York City, Inc. He has taught at the Columbia School of Social Work at Columbia University, and has guest lectured at the Silver School of Social Work at New York University.

Real change *is* possible

For more than fifty years, New Harbinger has published proven-effective self-help books and pioneering workbooks to help readers of all ages and backgrounds improve mental health and well-being, and achieve lasting personal growth. In addition, our spirituality books offer profound guidance for deepening awareness and cultivating healing, self-discovery, and fulfillment.

Founded by psychologist Matthew McKay and Patrick Fanning, New Harbinger is proud to be an independent, employee-owned company. Our books reflect our core values of integrity, innovation, commitment, sustainability, compassion, and trust. Written by leaders in the field and recommended by therapists worldwide, New Harbinger books are practical, accessible, and provide real tools for real change.

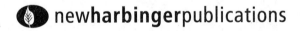 **newharbinger**publications

MORE BOOKS from
NEW HARBINGER PUBLICATIONS

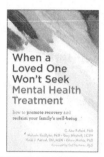

WHEN A LOVED ONE WON'T SEEK MENTAL HEALTH TREATMENT

How to Promote Recovery and Reclaim Your Family's Well-Being

978-1648483134 / US $19.95

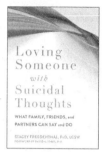

LOVING SOMEONE WITH SUICIDAL THOUGHTS

What Family, Friends, and Partners Can Say and Do

978-1648480249 / US $19.95

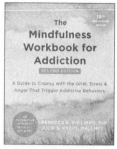

THE MINDFULNESS WORKBOOK FOR ADDICTION, SECOND EDITION

A Guide to Coping with the Grief, Stress, and Anger That Trigger Addictive Behaviors

978-1684038107 / US $24.95

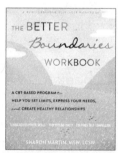

THE BETTER BOUNDARIES WORKBOOK

A CBT-Based Program to Help You Set Limits, Express Your Needs, and Create Healthy Relationships

978-1684037582 / US $24.95

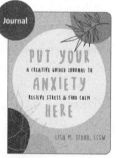

PUT YOUR ANXIETY HERE

A Creative Guided Journal to Relieve Stress and Find Calm

978-1648481451 / US $18.95

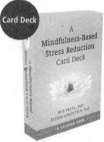

A MINDFULNESS-BASED STRESS REDUCTION CARD DECK

978-1684037797 / US $19.95

🌱 **newharbinger**publications

1-800-748-6273 / newharbinger.com

(VISA, MC, AMEX / prices subject to change without notice)

Follow Us 📷 👍 ✖ ▶ 📌 in ♪ 📧

Did you know there are **free tools** you can download for this book?

Free tools are things like **worksheets, guided meditation exercises**, and **more** that will help you get the most out of your book.

You can download free tools for this book— whether you bought or borrowed it, in any format, from any source—from the New Harbinger website. All you need is a NewHarbinger.com account. Just use the URL provided in this book to view the free tools that are available for it. Then, click on the "download" button for the free tool you want, and follow the prompts that appear to log in to your NewHarbinger.com account and download the material.

You can also save the free tools for this book to your **Free Tools Library** so you can access them again anytime, just by logging in to your account! Just look for this button on the book's free tools page.

+ Save this to my free tools library

If you need help accessing or downloading free tools, visit **newharbinger.com/faq** or contact us at **customerservice@newharbinger.com**.